£19.50

RIS

Perceptuo-motor
Difficulties

FORTHCOMING TITLES

Research Methods for Therapists
Avil Drummond

Group Work in Occupational Therapy
Linda Finlay

Stroke: Recovery and Rehabilitation
Polly Laidler

Caring for the Neurologically Damaged Adult
Ruth Nieuwenhuis

HIV and AIDS Care
S. Singh and L. Cusack

Speech and Language Disorders in Children
Dilys A. Treharne

Spinal Cord Rehabilitaiton
Karen Whalley-Hammell

THERAPY IN PRACTICE SERIES

Edited by Jo Campling

This series of books is aimed at 'therapists' concerned with rehabilitation in a very broad sense. The intended audience particularly includes occupational therapists, physiotherapists and speech therapists, but many titles will also be of interest to nurses, psychologists, medical staff, social workers, teachers or volunteer workers. Some volumes are interdisciplinary, others are aimed at one particular profession. All titles will be comprehensive but concise, and practical but with due reference to relevant theory and evidence. They are not research monographs but focus on professional practice, and will be of value to both students and qualified personnel.

Perceptuo-motor Difficulties :

Theory and strategies to help children, adolescents and adults

Dorothy E. Penso

Senior Occupational Therapist, Child Development Centre,
York District Hospital, York, UK

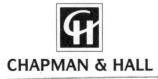

CHAPMAN & HALL

London · Glasgow · New York · Tokyo · Melbourne · Madras

Published by Chapman & Hall, 2–6 Boundary Row, London SE1 8HN

Chapman & Hall, 2–6 Boundary Row, London SE1 8HN, UK

Blackie Academic & Professional, Wester Cleddens Road, Bishopbriggs, Glasgow G64 2NZ, UK

Chapman & Hall, 29 West 35th Street, New York NY10001, USA

Chapman & Hall Japan, Thomson Publishing Japan, Hirakawacho Nemoto Building, 6F, 1-7-11 Hirakawa-cho, Chiyoda-ku, Tokyo 102, Japan

Chapman & Hall Australia, Thomas Nelson Australia, 102 Dodds Street, South Melbourne, Victoria 3205, Australia

Chapman & Hall India, R. Seshadri, 32 Second Main Road, CIT East, Madras 600 035, India

Distributed in the USA and Canada by Singular Publishing Group Inc., 4284 41st Street, San Diego, California 92105

First edition 1993

© 1993 Dorothy E. Penso

Typeset in 10/12 Palatino by Mews Photosetting, Beckenham, Kent
Printed in Great Britain by Page Bros, Norwich

ISBN 0 412 39810 9   1 56593 025 8 (USA)

A catalogue record for this book is available from the British Library

Contents

Acknowledgements

During my career as an occupational therapist I have met many children who have suffered from various perceptuo-motor difficulties. Their behaviour, and often very astute comments about areas of life in which they experienced problems, have provided much of my knowledge about these difficulties. Conversations with their parents and teachers have helped me to understand how these difficulties affect their relationships with family and peer groups. I would like to thank all these families for the insight with which they have provided me.

My thanks to the staff of the Postgraduate Library, York District Hospital and Mrs Kathy Crosbie, medical secretary for obtaining many of the papers to which I have referred.

I have appreciated the support of Jo Campling, commissioning editor, and the editorial staff of Chapman & Hall.

My husband, Giovanni, has supported and encouraged my writing with good humour and patience – thank you.

Figures 2.6 and 7.2 were drawn by Terry Winston.

Introduction

In the early years of this century a syndrome manifested by perceptuo-motor difficulties was described. During succeeding years further references were made to such a syndrome. In the first half of this century, however, children who suffered from such difficulties received little acknowledgement of their problems; few were neurologically assessed or offered remediation. Many school teachers were unaware of the existence of such problems and so were unable to make allowances for the gross and fine motor difficulties and perceptual problems encountered by some pupils during the course of the school day. Although many of these children were of average, and some of above average, ability, they were regarded as having little academic potential. Some were regarded as being 'educationally subnormal', a term applied at that time, because of perceptual problems which impaired reading ability and motor difficulties which affected their handwriting.

It was not until the 1960s that interest in the difficulties experienced by these children began to gather momentum. Paediatricians, therapists, teachers and psychologists became involved in research, assessment and treatment. Children began to be handled more sympathetically in school. Parents learned of the existence of such difficulties and sought help for their affected children. Today medics, paramedics and educationalists are consulting each other, sharing knowledge and expertise to the advantage of children with perceptuo-motor difficulties.

Some problems resolve with maturity, though a proportion of these children have difficulties which persist into adolescence. This is a period of life when there is supersensitivity to the comments and attitudes of peers and adults; it is a time when there is a strong desire to conform absolutely with the peer group. Adolescents who have perceptuo-motor difficulties often find these years particularly difficult.

Little medical or educational interest has been shown in the problems encountered during teenage years. Far less research has been undertaken than in children and little is offered by way of remediation or coping strategies. The problems of these adolescents may come to light when they are being investigated by psychologists or psychiatrists for emotional or personality difficulties. It may be that such difficulties occur in addition to perceptuo-motor ones or they may develop as a result of them.

Even less attention has been given to these problems when they are encountered during adult life. Those motor skills which are practised most often are most likely to improve, though many will continue to require conscious effort. Life skills often require consistent and continuing effort, a fact often overlooked by family, friends and even medical and paramedical practitioners.

Perceptuo-motor difficulties can present lifelong problems. They affect every aspect of life: posture and gesture, motor and motor planning skills, visual and auditory perception. They influence relationships with other people, the activities of daily living, educational, vocational and leisure pursuits.

This book reviews investigations and research undertaken to discover the nature of perceptuo-motor problems of childhood, considers remedial programmes and strategies which have been employed. It discusses the problems of the child whose difficulties persist throughout childhood.

The greater part of the book, however, is concerned with the perceptuo-motor difficulties of adolescence and adult life which, to date, have received comparatively little attention. Many adolescents and adults experience considerable difficulty with skills which are performed with little conscious thought or active effort by the majority of the population; posture and personal appearance, choosing and sustaining an appropriate career, coping with domestic and child-care activities, leisure pursuits and hobbies. Suggestions are made of effective ways to undertake activities – from applying make-up and caring for hair to taking a photograph and swallowing a tablet.

This book does not consider specifically perceptuo-motor difficulties which are acquired as the result of head injury, cerebrovascular accident or acquired neurological disease. Some of the strategies and techniques described may, however, be helpful in such conditions. It will provide insight into perceptuo-motor problems for medical and paramedical staff who are perhaps treating clients for other unrelated problems, in particular, physiotherapists, occupational therapists, speech and language therapists and orthoptists. Teachers and lecturers in secondary, tertiary and adult education will find that an understanding and appreciation of the effects of perceptuo-motor difficulties will alert them to the possibility of a proportion of their students experiencing them and enable them to adopt a constructive and sympathetic attitude towards them. Training, career and personnel officers will be alert to the possibility of such difficulties in their clients and thus staff will be able to plan appropriate training and give realistic career advice.

Clinical, educational and occupational psychologists will be aware of the effects of perceptuo-motor difficulties on 'body language', appearance, motor skills and even emotional responses. They will also be aware that such problems can also have effects on the manner and speed with which written tests are completed. People with perceptuo-motor difficulties often show a significant discrepancy between verbal and performance scores of psychological tests.

It is important that anyone who comes into contact with people, professionally or socially, should be aware of the effects of perceptuo-motor difficulties. That really means that each one of us should be aware of the effects of such difficulties; thus much misunderstanding of gestures, actions and emotional response could be avoided. Allowances will then be made in activities which these people find difficult to accomplish and their positive skills will be appreciated and used to the benefit of society in general. In addition, the satisfaction, self-esteem and motivation of those who suffer from perceptuo-motor difficulties will be enhanced.

1

Perceptuo-motor difficulties in children – theory and remediation

Not so much a syndrome – more a way of life.
Dr Ian McKinlay, 1987

For many generations there have been children who were described as, 'butter fingers', 'all fingers and thumbs' or 'His fingers are all thumbs' (Brewer, 1978). Children have been told to 'put their tongue away' when it has been protruded during some intricate fine motor task and was mirroring the movements of the hands. 'Wipe your mouth', children have been told as they drooled while applying themselves to an exacting task. Countless young people have been described as having 'two left feet', as being 'too slow to catch cold' of 'looking awkward' when observed performing some complex gross or fine motor task. Such children will almost certainly have been described as 'clumsy' on more than one occasion. 'Clumsy' is a word derived from Norwegian, *klummsen*, which means benumbed, which is pretty much how some such children must feel when attempting some complex tasks or practising precise skills.

It appears that the general population was well aware of children who suffered from perceptuo-motor difficulties long before the medical and paramedical professions gave their attention to the problems. Such difficulties were not analysed or appreciated as being of a motor or perceptual nature but were accepted as innate characteristics of the person concerned. Treatment or remediation was not considered in relation to these difficulties, for 'clumsiness' or 'awkwardness' was not considered to be a 'medical' or 'treatable' problem.

WHY DO SOME PEOPLE SEEM TO BE 'CLUMSY'?

Mention was first made at the beginning of this century of the 'motor deficiency' from which some people appeared to suffer. Descriptions such as 'congenitally maladroit' and 'awkwardness of movement' were also used. Children were examined and described as having exaggerated tendon reflexes, mild hypertonicity and associated movements. Emphasis was on the signs which were observed or could be elicited. Orton was, perhaps, the first to mention symptoms other than those of motor effect. He attributed these signs to disorders of praxis and gnosis. These early investigations are described by Hulme and Lord (1986) in their paper 'Clumsy children – a review of recent research'.

In order to understand and, hence, remediate so called perceptuo-motor difficulties, much more than motor activity must be considered. Motor activity, except reflex actions, requires motor planning or praxis which is preceded by a further mental activity, perception. This perception is, perforce, of sensation either from within self or from the environment. Thus, if there is a deficit in any link of this chain of events, behaviour may appear to be uncoordinated or 'clumsy' (see Figure 1.1).

Sensory information may be provided by any of the sense organs, the eyes, the ears, the olfactory apparatus of the nose, the taste buds of the tongue or the tactile receptors in the skin. Sensory information about the position of the body is provided by proprioception, the awareness of posture, balance and position provided by receptors in muscles, tendons and joints in addition to information provided by vestibular apparatus of the inner ear.

Straightforward deficits of visual and auditory acuity are usually reasonably easily diagnosed. Other deficits such as imperfect visual convergence, diminished tactile sensation or poor proprioceptive abilities may be more difficult to detect.

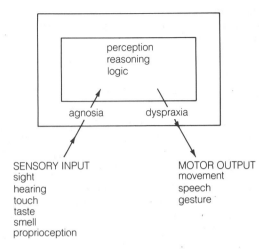

Figure 1.1 Diagrammatic representation of the chain of events from sensory input to motor output, illustrating the points at which the process may be impaired.

Before sensory information may be perceived it must be recognized. For example a face must be recognized as such. Inability to do so is known as agnosia and is attributed to a disturbance of the association area of the cerebral cortex.

Perception of sensory information can also be described in lay terms such as common sense, understanding, 'nous'. It is the ability to appreciate the qualities of information transmitted by the organs of sensation, to make sense of the environment and people and objects within it. Perception at a basic level involves making sense of shape, size, colour, the relationships of objects to each other and to self. It also includes more complex abilities such as form constancy, appreciating an object from whichever angle it is viewed, and figure–background discrimination. The latter skill is necessary at a gross level to be able to concentrate on an appropriate visual or auditory stimulus in an environment which is presenting a number of stimuli. For example in a lecture hall there may be the sound of students' pens moving across note pads, pages being turned, the whirr of the motor of an overhead projector, the creaks of doors opening and closing in an adjacent corridor, yet students for most the time will have little difficulty giving their attention to the words of the lecturer. At a fine level the person who has difficulty with figure–background discrimination may have problems picking out the appropriate line from a whole printed page.

Sensory input and perception of that input usually results in some form of motor output. Sensory input could be described as stimulus and motor output as response. In order for that motor response to be made, unless it is a reflex action, it must be planned. Motor planning or praxis is frequently an area of difficulty and one which is difficult to remediate, for to be effective the motor planning element of a skill must be accomplished without conscious effort. Perhaps the most complex skill which requires precise motor planning is handwriting. The hand holding the pen must trace exact, small and different shapes while concentration is given to the content of the writing. In recent years many children with such difficulties have been helped by using a keyboard to record words on paper. A keyboard removes the need to plan the shape of each letter character so that the necessary concentration may be given to the content of the piece of work.

Perceptuo-motor difficulties may result from many and varied causes. Consideration of the chain of events from sensory input to motor output will aid diagnosis and provide starting points on which to base treatment.

It was not until the late 1960s that there began to be a positive interest in the nature of symptoms suffered by these children. It was at this time that interest was shown not only in the examination of these children, in order to elicit the nature of their difficulties, but also in the development of treatment programmes.

> The purpose of this paper is to emphasize that children with visuo-motor disabilities are often in need of special help, and that this must be given at an early age if secondary emotional and behaviour disorders are to be prevented.
> Dare and Gordon, 1970

RETROSPECTIVE REPORTS OF EARLY DIFFICULTIES

A number of studies of children with perceptuo-motor difficulties have looked back at their previous history, very often as reported by parents. In a group of 15 children described as clumsy, nine parents reported problems in more than two areas. Eleven of the children had or continue to have problems associated with speech or hearing. One child had been 'very small for dates' and had dysmorphic features (Henderson and Hall, 1982).

Retrospectively, problems experienced by children early in life, seem to be common amongst those who later prove to suffer from perceptuo-motor difficulties. Parents of 32 children with motor/learning difficulties who attended an occupational therapy department over a 2-year period were interviewed to explore their psychosocial and physiological early development (Stephenson, McKay and Chesson 1990). Eighteen parents reported that their child had had perinatal problems; twelve of the children had spent some time in a special care baby unit; one third of the children were reported to have had initial feeding or weaning difficulties. Sixteen of the children had not crawled before beginning to walk. More than half the parents reported that their child had had speech difficulties, the exact type of which is not stated. We cannot therefore know if the problems were of a receptive or expressive nature or, in fact, if the problems were purely articulatory or of a more central nature. Nine of the children had been referred to the regional child development unit before the age of 2 years. The same number had had speech therapy before the age of 3.5 years. Difficulties with toilet training were reported by 45% of the parents.

A recent study of children of very low birth-weight showed that they had 'significantly higher Impairment Scores' than their matched controls when tested on the Test of Motor Impairment (TOMI). The very low birth-weight children were also perceived to be more overactive and more easily frightened than the controls. Their teachers also perceived them as being more fidgety (Roberts, Marlow and Cooke, 1989),

Dare and Gordon (1970) describe a high incidence of complications in the perinatal period, including the effects of eclampsia and bleeding during pregnancy, short gestation, birth asphyxia, epilepsy in the neonatal period, icterus neonatorum, episodes of cyanosis and concussion. This high incidence of perinatal complications was also found by

Johnston, Short and Crawford (1987) in their study of 95 poorly coordinated children in Adelaide, Australia.

INCIDENCE

Attempts to identify the percentage of the population who suffer from perceptuo-motor difficulties is complicated in a number of ways.

1. Criteria for diagnosing a child as 'clumsy' or suffering from perceptuo-motor difficulties are not clear-cut. Paediatricians, for instance, may use different measurement scales from therapists and educational psychologists may look at these children from yet another angle. Thus different studies would conclude that differing percentages of their subjects should be included in the category.
2. Some parents are more ready than others to seek advice should they suspect such difficulties in their child.
3. Teachers too, vary in the acuteness of their observations of the motor and perceptual skills of their pupils. They may view such difficulties as being the result of previous inappropriate teaching methods or lack of practice.
4. Many research projects study a highly selected group of subjects and so their results do not indicate prevalence in the general population.

Results of studying children who have been assessed as being 'clumsy', or as having perceptuo-motor difficulties, can lead to the deduction that the proportion of such children must be at least that suggested by the study and that it is highly likely that the percentage will be considerably higher.

In a recent study of 400 children, aged between 5 and 8 years, 20 (5%) were found to have motor impairment severe enough to affect their progress in school (Henderson and Hall, 1982). In another study with a cohort of 200 children, with a mean age of 5.6 years, 8.5% were identified as 'clumsy'. The authors comment that this is a higher proportion than has been found in other studies and suggest that this may be because of the early age at which the children were tested (Roussounis, Gaussen and Stratton, 1987).

Should these percentages prove to be realistic, there would be at least one child in every classroom who suffers from this type of difficulty. Should the problems not resolve spontaneously or be successfully treated, there must be an average of at least one sufferer riding on every bus. Every theatre audience will include at least a dozen. The problem is large, not least for individual people with these problems.

Interestingly, people of many professions who work with these children have found that the number of boys who are referred to them greatly exceeds the number of girls (Table 1.1).

Table 1.1 Numbers of boys and girls in various studies

Boys	Girls	Study
13	3	Losse *et al.*, 1991
29	2	Stevenson, McKay and Chesson, 1990
33	9	Gillberg, Gillberg and Groth, 1989
31	9	Laszlo, Bairstow and Bartrip, 1988
18	8	Knuckey and Gubbay, 1983
13	3	Henderson and Hall, 1982
16	3	Dare and Gordon, 1970

WHAT ARE THE SYMPTOMS OF PERCEPTUO-MOTOR IMPAIRED CHILDREN?

The range of characteristics attributed to children with perceptuo-motor difficulties is diverse. It probably depends to some extent on the professional interests of researchers. Hulme and Lord (1986) described four core features:

1. Impaired motor performance of a degree sufficient to interfere seriously with many activities essential to daily life.
2. Absence or relative paucity of (hard) neurological signs.
3. Normal or near normal intellectual capacity.
4. Discrepancies in motor capacity, with relative dexterity being exhibited in some motor activities and gross impairment in others.

Dare and Gordon (1970) described three subgroups of children within the group who attended outpatient clinics of the Children's Hospital in Manchester. The first and largest subgroup was described as suffering from a 'specific development disorder', a second group as having 'general retarded development' and a third as suffering from 'minimal cerebral palsy'.

Henderson and Hall (1982) also divided their subjects into three groups, 'the first included the academically successful children whose motor impairment was an isolated disability . . . the second group included those at the low end of the ability scale, often with considerable social and behavioural disorders, for whom clumsiness was merely one of many problems. The third group could be regarded as an intermediate group and perhaps would be less likely that the other two to attract medical or educational attention.'

WHAT ARE THE CONCOMITANTS OF PERCEPTUO-MOTOR IMPAIRMENT?

There are many other features which commonly occur together with perceptuo-motor difficulties. Often it is not clear whether these characteristics present in addition to perceptuo-motor ones or develop as a result of them. The school career of many of these children is fraught with disappointment and frustration. Many manifest emotional and behavioural problems, they are easily distracted by the noise and movements of other activities in the classroom, have rapid mood swings and display uninhibited behaviour. It would be reasonable to deduce that these behaviours are a result of difficulties experienced because of perceptuo-motor problems. This, however need not be so; these behaviours may occur together with perceptuo-motor symptoms but may not be dependent on them. Frequently there is continuing speech and hearing difficulty (Henderson and Hall, 1982; Johnston, Short and Crawford, 1987).

IS THE PROBLEM MORE THAN ONE OF PERCEPTUO-MOTOR DIFFICULTIES?

Care should be taken when assessing and treating these children for, very occasionally, their problems are much more serious than is initially apparent. Some degenerative neurological conditions present, in the early stages, as uncomplicated perceptuo-motor difficulties. Very occasionally early symptoms of more serious conditions may be those of poor motor coordination or delayed development of motor skills. One of the reasons for this is that children are in the process of acquiring skills of an increasingly finer nature. For example, children are not expected to begin to write until they are 4 or 5 years old. They are 5 or 6 years old before it is expected that they will be able to tie shoe-laces. Pre-school children are usually allowed a great deal of choice in the types of play in which they will take part. Parents usually accept, for instance, the choice of their child who 'prefers' to dig in the garden than draw with crayons. Few parents would question their child's choice of play or associate it with any specific problem. It is therefore all too easy for early symptoms of neurological conditions to pass undetected in young children.

Case note

As five years of age, Ian presented as a clumsy child with slight ataxia. In retrospect his parents realized that he had never been as agile as his peers. His parents were first to notice deterioration in his motor skills. His ataxia increased, his speech became slightly less distinct, he developed a slight kyphosis and tight tendo-Achilles. Further investigations were undertaken which resulted in the diagnosis of Friedreich's ataxia, an inherited, progressive condition.

Assessments of children who are suspected of having perceptuo-motor difficulties should always be undertaken and observations recorded with great care so that it is possible to compare performances on different occasions. Even this does not remove the possiblity of missing subtle changes in ability. Firstly, children in a test situation, however discreetly this is arranged, will usually perform at their optimum level which cannot possibly be sustained throughout everyday life. Secondly, where the record of performance is a written one, it is difficult to describe in sufficient detail the *quality* of performance. A record of quality of movement and skill performance is far more significant than one which simply notes success or failure. If performance is to be recorded sequentially, a description of quality will be a more sensitive tool than a ticked checklist. With the former, subtle changes in performance will be measurable and deterioration noted. A checklist will only provide information of what a child can and cannot do and provide little information which will enable the assessor to deduce the reasons for success or failure.

SHOULD ALL CHILDREN WHO ARE DIAGNOSED AS HAVING PERCEPTUO-MOTOR DIFFICULTIES BE TREATED?

Children who have been singled out for diagnosis and assessment must have been observed to have difficulty in at least one area of life. As the realities of perceptuo-motor problems become better known, both by professionals and the general population, more children are having their motor and perceptual abilities assessed and in many cases treatment programmes are offered.

Children with the most severe difficulties are often diagnosed in their pre-school years. Others are found to have difficulties upon school entry. The difficulties of some children may not become obvious until they are required to produce large amounts of swift and legible handwriting, and accomplish other fine motor and precise gross motor skills with speed and without conscious effort.

Whether all these groups of children should be assessed and treated is arguable. The following points need to be considered.

1. A number of studies have suggested that at least 5% of the child population suffers from some degree of such difficulties (Henderson and Hall, 1982; Roussounis, Gaussen and Stratton, 1987). Would it be realistic to fund the resources to make a detailed assessment and administer prolonged treatment programmes to this large number of children? Should the aim be to assess all potentially clumsy children and treat only those with the severest problems? Who would judge the severity of the problems; a medical consultant, a therapist, the child's parents or teachers?

2. For some children and their families, the process of assessment and sympathetic explanation of the nature of the problem to the child, parents and teachers has proved to be effective, at least in the short term (Roussounis, Gaussen and Stratton, 1987). Parents are relieved to learn that there are reasons for their child's shortcomings. An explanation of the nature of the difficulties, related to the actual skills with which the child has difficulty, will often relieve

stress and tension within the family. All children behave at times in ways which cause handling difficulties, but it is likely that difficult behaviour is more often caused by difficulties with sensory input, perception and/or motor planning and motor output. A discussion along such lines will often defuse potentially explosive situations.

Many children have been greatly helped by having their difficulties explained to them in a manner appropriate to their age and understanding. The honest assurance that such difficulties do not detract from the child's value as a person, from being a likeable child or from intellectual ability at whatever level that may be, boosts the child's self-image and self-esteem. Teachers must also be made aware of the nature of the child's difficulties for it is often in an educational setting that such difficulties are most prominent.

3. The decision regarding treatment also depends on the child's own attitudes to self and the skills which are personally important; these will depend on age. It is easier and often more effective to treat a child during infant or early junior school years, than later when self-consciousness and embarrassment often inhibit cooperation in remedial programmes.

Case note

Neil, a 7-year-old boy, was referred for assessment and possible treatment by an occupational therapist. Assessment showed that he had moderately severe difficulties with motor planning at both a gross and fine motor level. He was an academically inclined child and was enthusiastic about a programme to improve his handwriting skills.

He was less enthusiastic about help with his gross motor skills. He expressed his reasons for this attitude thus. 'We only have a games lesson twice a week, so I can manage that. I need to write every day. My best friend is the best in our class at games but I'm the best reader.' His therapist respected his point of view and concentrated treatment on improving handwriting skills.

Neil mastered the art of swift, legible handwriting, a skill which he considered to be important but was happy to accept his difficulties with games and gymnastics; they were not important to him. He is now 13 years old, making excellent academic progress. He is a well adjusted boy who is popular with his peers despite having little hope or desire to be a star in the gymnasium or on the sports field.

4. For some children periods of specific treatment are important and, in some cases, vital if the child is to learn to function satisfactorily in many areas of life. The nature of the treatment which is offered will depend, to some extent, on the types of treatment which are being offered in the area in which the child lives. This, in turn, will be affected by the treatment systems which are in vogue at the time and the philosophies of the therapists concerned. How long any type of treatment needs to be continued is yet to be proven. Improvement has been claimed in the short term for many treatment techniques. Children have been reported to have 'improved', though such a vague term could be a subjective opinion of the therapist concerned. Because many treatment techniques have been developed only in recent years it is not possbile to evaluate their long-term effects.

TREATMENT PROGRAMMES

Remediation of perceptuo-motor problems is based broadly upon two basic concepts.

The activity-based approach

The actual activities in which the child is demonstrating difficulty are practised. This approach relies on the belief that repeated practise of a skill will result in the improved execution of that skill. Usually such activities are broken down into a number of smaller skills, each being taught and practised separately. In this type of approach, equipment, the environment and the activities chosen to be taught would be selected and, if necessary adapted, according to the needs of the child.

The function-based approach

The therapist concentrates on the underlying functional abilities which are necessary to accomplish specific activities, not on activities themselves. A child who is found to have kinesthetic deficit is trained in this function and not in the activities in which that function is necessary. A child who had spatial difficulties would be trained in that particular function in the belief that this underlying ability would then be successfully incorporated into activities of which it is a component. This approach assumes that these functions can be taught and that if this is true, and they are learned in a therapeutic situation, they will then be generalized and incorporated into the activities of childhood.

DEVELOPMENTAL TESTS

The first steps in assessment may involve the use of developmental norms (Frankenburg and Dodds, 1969; Sheridan, 1975; Illingworth, 1983). Measuring the abilities of a child against that of the so-called average, gives some indication of in what way and by how much a child's performance deviates from that 'average' level. When using such scales, it is important to appreciate the wide range of patterns of development which fall within normal limits. It is also important to appreciate that the performance of the child with perceptuo-motor difficulties may be affected in many areas not directly associated with these types of difficulty. For example, a child may be asked to build a bridge with three 2.5 cm wooden cubes. The child may understand the relative positions of the bricks which compose the bridge and have the motor skill to hold, place and release the cubes. The child may, however, fail to construct a bridge because of problems with motor planning.

It is not sufficient to discover whether or not a child is able to accomplish certain motor and perceptual skills and to compare performance with the results of tests which have been standardized on large populations of children. This type of testing will be profitable only if further questions are asked. Which abilities and skills does the child possess which have led to success in a particular task? Which skills and abilities does the child lack which have prevented the accomplishment of a particular activity?

A number of treatment programmes have been developed which are intended to enhance various deficient functional skills. They have been implemented by therapists of various disciplines. One of the best known is Frostig's (1966) Test of Visual Perception. The tests have been standardizd for children between 3.5 and 8.0 years of age. It is suggested that those whose perceptual quotient (PQ) falls below 90 using the Frostig's test, are in need of remediation because, it is asserted, below this score children are unlikely to learn to read, especially if taught mainly by visual methods.

A study has been described (Maslow, Frostig, Lefever and Whittlesey, 1963) in which children who fell below this score either entered a training programme devised by Frostig and Horne (1964) or remained in their normal classroom situation. Both groups of children were then re-tested using the same test material. Both groups had improved their performance 'but the trained group gained significantly more' (Maslow, Frostig, Lefever and Whittlesey, 1963). The test and subsequent treatment programme rely on the basic assumptions the test really does test the functions it is intended to test, that these functions are necessary for academic progress and that deficit in these functions does respond to treatment. There is also the possibility that the training programme trains children successfully to complete the test rather than improve the functions in which they have been diagnosed as deficient.

The importance of 'sensory integration' is the basis of Jean Ayres' assessment and treatment techniques. 'It is postulated that the increased integration of sensory input from the body . . . enhances the ability to perceive and associate visual and auditory stimuli' (Ayres, 1974). Jean Ayres states that 'if a human being cannot perform purposeful acts, in the sense that a predetermined goal can be reached, all the muscular strength and integration of upper motor neuron function will be to little avail.' The process which is necessary for these 'purposeful acts' to take place requires sensory receptors to be stimulated and these impulses to be transmitted to the central nervous system. Sensory information must then be organized and interpreted, in other words perceived. Motor activity takes place, in many instances as a response to perception. Development of perceptual skills is further reinforced by sensory feedback from motor activity.

Jean Ayres describes four major sensory areas which contribute to perception which precede motor planning and motor execution: touch, proprioception, vestibular function and vision. The Southern California Motor Accuracy Test (Ayres, 1972) is designed to measure the degree and changes in sensorimotor integration and to assist in the diagnosis of perceptuo-motor dysfunction.

Suggested treatment of diagnosed deficits is multi-sensory, following a developmental sequence. Ayres stresses the need to develop very basic perceptions such as awareness of the configuration of the body and coordination of the two sides of the body. Tactile and vestibular stimulation is used and emphasis is given to the development of equilibrium reaction.

More recent studies have pinpointed the importance of kinesthesis on motor behaviour.

> Kinethesis is the sense which conveys information about the position of the body and limbs; about the direction and extent of movement; the speed of movement; and the force the muscles exert. There are two further areas in which kinesthesis is necessary in skilled motor performance. Firstly, to perform a movement smoothly and accurately one must detect errors in the course of the movement, to make corrections possible. Errors are sensed kinesthetically. Secondly, one remembers the feel of movements but does not remember which muscles were moved. That is memory for movements is stored kinesthetically.
>
> Laszlo, Bairstow and Bartrip, 1988

Kinethesis is thought to be a basic process, the teaching of which opens the way to the learning of complex skills. There are many other systems of evaluating sensory, perceptual and motor competence, some being medically-based and others having an underlying educational approach. A review of these various approaches is provided in *The Assessment of 'Clumsy' Children: Old and New Approaches* (Henderson, 1987).

Much research has been undertaken into the efficacy of various types of remedial programmes following assessment which has highlighted areas of difficulty. Evaluation of treatment programmes has produced encouraging results, reporting improved abilities in the child involved. It is, however, difficult to find reports of the long-term effects of these programmes. For example, do adolescents who had some form or treatment for perceptual deficit in childhood, function better than a group who had no treatment? That is, how long-lasting are the effects of treatment?

2

Understanding the effects of perceptuo-motor difficulties of childhood

Boys and girls come out to play,
The moon doth shine as bright as day.
Leave your supper and leave your sleep,
And join your playfellows in the street.

English nursery rhyme

There is no panacea for perceptuo-motor difficulties; they are complex and varying in nature. No programme designed to remediate perceptuo-motor problems has been proved to be a permanent 'cure' for them. Until such a programme is available there will be children who will need help to overcome or circumvent their difficulties. Explanation and discussion will help the child concerned and provide insight into specific difficulties which will enable parents, teachers and others involved with the child to understand and offer constructive help.

The activities of childhood may be divided in three broad areas; Personal independence according to developmental level, play and leisure activities, and formal education.

INDEPENDENCE ACTIVITIES

Many parents will welcome an explanation of the causes of the difficulties their child is experiencing with accomplishing a particular task or activity, together with suggestions of strategies and devices they can introduce into daily life to facilitate activities and ease any stress which such problems may cause.

Eating and drinking

Often the parents of children who experience perceptuo-motor difficulties will comment upon one of two problems concerning eating and drinking; faddiness regarding the items of food the child will eat and general messiness when eating or drinking. Some parents complain of their child's difficulties in both these areas.

Faddy eating habits

A child may develop faddy eating habits for a number of reasons, all of which must considered before it may be concluded that the problem is due solely to perceptuo-motor difficulties. A discussion between the child and his/her parents will usually clarify the situation.

Children are not completely free agents about what is included in their diets. By the time children are born, their parents will have a well-established dietary pattern which they will adhere to when feeding their children. Many spouses will indulge their partner's food fads, eliminating unfavoured items of food from their diet. Thus all members of the family may be offered a very limited diet.

Parents differ in the amount of skill they have in preparing meals and the degree of interest and enthusiasm they have in eating it. In some homes a minimum of time is spent preparing, presenting and eating food. Mealtimes are not anticipated with pleasure and the children of such families do not see their parents enjoying their meal. Thus, they too fail to develop enthusiasm for the events as pleasurable family occasions.

Children manipulate adults if they are allowed to do so. Parents are often very anxious to ensure that their children take a diet sufficient in quantity and nutrition. During the first year of life infants eat more in proportion to their body-weight than they will do for the rest of their lives. Having become accustomed to this relatively large intake of food during the first year, many parents find it difficult in subsequent years, to assess the amount their children should eat. Parents may resort to coaxing their children to eat what they consider to be an adequate diet which may be larger than the child needs or is able to eat. Children can be deterred from eating by over-filled plates. Children can also sense their parents anxiety and may refuse food in order to manipulate them.

Case note

By the age of 10 years David ate only a very limited diet, consisting of chips, beefburgers, fish fingers, peas, apple pie and icecream. He had been a 'small for dates' baby who was very irritable during his early days. His weight gain was poor. As he began to eat a solid diet, his mother was understandably anxious that he ate well. She resorted to coaxing and cajoling him in her attempts to ensure that he took an adequate diet. David was quick to sense his mother's concern and anxiety at mealtimes. He used food refusal to manipulate her. Before very long she was cooking one meal for the rest of the family and items from this limited diet for David.

It was not until David became independent and lived alone that his diet became more varied. Had his taste in food changed or was there now little point in maintaining his 'special' diet now that there was no one there to be concerned about it?

It is important therefore to ascertain whether the eating problem is of a perceptuo-motor or behavioural nature. The problem may, of course, be a mixture of both types of difficulty.

Physical difficulties with eating

Some children who have perceptuo-motor difficulties enjoy a limited diet because of physical difficulties with chewing and swallowing food. Listening to a parent's account of what foods their child chooses to eat and what is refused will not only provide an indication of their child's diet but will also indicate the types of food which have been offered to the child.

The child who has physical difficulty with handling food in the mouth will usually avoid fibrous items such as roast meats, vegetables (except peas, baked beans and potatoes) nuts and unpeeled fruit and many items of salad. They will usually find highly processed foods acceptably because any fibrous content will have been reduced to pulp. Items such as biscuits and potato crisps which will melt or disintegrate when mixed with saliva will also be acceptable. Thus many children with such difficuties will enjoy eating biscuits, crisps, bread, pastry, cakes, fishcakes, minced meat but will avoid roast beef, unpeeled apples, green leafy vegetables, celery and other fibrous vegetables.

Children who seem to have an aversion to fibrous food may have a poor chewing pattern, that is, they have not developed rotary chewing but move their jaw only up and down and mash food with their tongue. They are in fact attempting to mash their food rather than grind it. Grinding is particularly important for effective mastication of meat. Children with these problems will often find that meat which is even a little tough will be chewed and chewed, ineffectively, and become a stringy tasteless bolus which they are unable to swallow.

Once parents and the child involved understand the problem they will have gone a long way towards solving it. The child will be relieved to know that their problem is acknowledged and there is understanding that their food preferences are not only the result of being 'naughty' or difficult. (This is not to suggest that children with chewing difficulties cannot at times also behave badly at mealtimes including refusing to eat some types of food.) Parents will understand why their child prefers not to eat certain foods and thus anxiety at mealtimes will be reduced.

Improving chewing patterns

To enable more effective chewing, as well as sociable eating habits, the child should be encouraged to chew food with the mouth closed. It is not possible to chew properly with the mouth open. The child may not be aware of chewing without the lips together and attention will need to be drawn to maintaining lip closure. Initially eating whilst looking in a mirror will help the child to ensure lip closure whilst chewing. Sitting position is important when it is considered that lip closure is facilitated when the neck is flexed but more difficult when the neck is extended. Initially lip closure whilst chewing can also be encouraged by gentle hand pressure under the lower jaw. Rotary chewing may then be encouraged by gently moving the child's lower jaw in rotary fashion until the action has been learned.

Both chewing patterns and gagging may be affected by the amount of food taken into the mouth at any one time. Inability to use a knife and fork effectively can lead to the child putting too much food into the mouth at once. The child who has difficulty cutting meat for instance may choose to put an overlarge piece into the mouth. Problems with chewing may not, therefore, be confined to the mechanics of chewing but also involve difficulty with manipulating cutlery. Putting appropriately sized pieces of food into the mouth may also be impeded by lack of judgement of size and mismatching the size of pieces of food with the appropriate amount which can be comfortably taken into the mouth and chewed.

The child's experience of using cutlery

It should not be assumed that all families eat whilst sitting at a table. The diet of some families consists of a series of snacks, held in the hand and eaten on the move. Children of such families will have little experience of using cutlery.

Many families choose to balance a plate on their knees while sitting in an easy chair. This is not the best position for a child to learn to use a knife and fork. A child who would have had only slight delay in learning to manipulate cutlery sitting on a suitable chair at a table may have had considerable difficulty learning to do so eating from a plate balanced on the lap.

Even if a family always eats whilst sitting at a table, sometimes little account is taken of the length of a child's trunk in relationship to the height of the chair seat and the height of the table. For the child who has difficulty learning to use cutlery it is an additional problem if the table is at shoulder height! Parents attention should be drawn to the possibility of this additional difficulty and suggestions made in keeping with the family's lifestyle of how the child may be more appropriately seated.

For some children their first experience of using a knife and fork may be when they eat school dinner. Not all parents consider the use of cutlery to be an important skill to teach their children. In some homes much of the food which is given to children is held in the hand or eaten with fingers from a plate. Always consider the possibility of lack of experience as a reason for a child not being able to handle cutlery effectively.

Transferring food from plate to mouth

In order to be able to transfer food by means of a fork or spoon into the mouth the child must know exactly where the mouth is, usually without visual monitoring. This is an obvious statement but it must be remembered that many children who suffer from perceptuo-motor difficulties have problems with body image, their own position in space and the relationships of the various parts of their body to each other. A conscious effort may be required to transfer each mouthful successfully from plate to mouth. For the majority of people who eat without conscious effort or thought this can be a difficult concept to understand. As with all other motor activities, eating for the child with perceptuo-motor difficulties may require constant conscious effort.

Added to these problems are often difficulties with maintaining concentration, and distractibility. Should a child be distracted by an unexpected noise or movement the head may be turned away from the loaded fork or spoon as it is moved towards the mouth.

Handling cutlery

The ways in which cutlery is used varies according to the food being eaten and the customs of particular societies. Many British people when eating a traditional meal of roast meat and vegetables will use a fork in the left hand and a knife in the right. Thus food is being transferred to the mouth using, for a high proportion of people, the non-preferred hand. This custom dates back to the days when only a knife was used for eating, first for cutting food and then transferring it to the mouth. It was not until the 16th century that the fork began to gain in popularity and be used for transferring food to the mouth. The knife had always been held in the right hand and so forks are traditionally held in the left (Hayward, 1957).

People in many parts of the USA will cut up the food on their plate then lay the knife on the side of the plate, transfer the fork to the right hand and continue to eat using only the fork.

The Italian diet which contains a large proportion of pasta and rice dishes usually use only a fork held in the preferred, usually the right hand. (There is still prejudice amongst some Italians against being a left-handed person, *un mancino*). A piece of bread held in the non-preferred hand is sometimes used to help food on to the fork.

Children who need to visually monitor their hand movements will find handling a piece of cutlery in each hand difficult; it is impossible to monitor the movements of both hands simultaneously. Such children may take longer than average to master handling a knife and fork or fork and spoon. They will need help and understanding of their difficulties. Some families believe that eating using two pieces of cutlery is an important social skill. Some parents insist that the fork is held in the left hand and the knife in the right. Whilst it is not the therapists role to criticize or try to alter the lifestyle or philosophies of their clients, in the case of the child who has continuing difficulty with handling cutlery it is reasonable to explain the nature of such difficulties and suggest simplified methods of using cutlery which are both effective and socially acceptable.

For those who have a more able left than right hand, changing the knife to the left hand and the fork to the right whilst cutting up food will be helpful. Where the reverse situation appertains it may help to transfer the fork to the right hand whilst it is being used to transfer food from plate to mouth. Similarly when using a fork and spoon the more able hand should hold the piece of cutlery which is used to transfer the food to the mouth.

Cutting food

Many people who have perceptuo-motor difficulties find cutting food difficult. Parents often complain that their child is a 'messy eater' and that 'at the end of a meal there is always food on the table'. It is important that the child is provided with a knife which is capable of cutting food! That is not to suggest that the child should have a knife which is razor sharp but one that has an effective cutting edge. Sometimes parents of a child who they consider to be clumsy feel that a knife capable of cutting would be dangerous in their child's hand.

Such a child needs to be taught that the knife does the cutting and that cutting food does not depend on the degree of pressure they exert upon the knife. Many children will attempt to pull the food apart rather than cut it. To demonstrate an effective cutting movement the adult should place a hand over the child's hand on the knife and proceed to move the knife back and forth until the food is cut. Thus the child will learn the necessary movement and will be able to feel the degree of pressure which is most effective.

Choice of cutlery

Much modern cutlery is designed entirely in stainless steel, the handles of which (in keeping with the design of the pieces) are very slim. Such handles can be difficult to grip firmly, particularly by those who suffer from perceptuo-motor diffi-culties. Cutlery with chunkier handles is usually easier to grip effectively. Cutlery is available with wood, bone or plastic handles. Handles which provide the most friction, those with matt surfaces, are perhaps the most suitable.

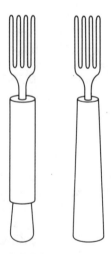

Figure 2.1 Cutlery with enlarged handles to facilitate a secure grip. A piece of foam rubber tubing has been fitted to the handle of the fork on the left. The fork on the right is of the type which may be purchased with an enlarged handle already fitted.

It may be helpful, as a temporary measure, to enlarge handles by the addition of foam tubing which will increase the diameter of the handle and also provide a resiliant matt gripping surface. Cutlery with enlarged handles is commercially available (Figure 2.1 and Appendix B).

Crockery

A plate which has a slight lip will help to prevent food slipping from the plate. This is not to suggest that a child should be provided with a plate or dish which is inappropriate to her/his age.

Cups, beakers and tumblers which are straight-sided are less easily tipped over than ones which taper towards the bottom. Shallow, dumpy drinking vessels are easier to handle and drink from than tall narrow ones.

A place-mat made from non-slip material, such as Dycem, helps to stabilize crockery.

Checklist for use with children who appear to have feeding difficulties

1. Is it really a feeding problem?
   (a) Is the child a faddy eater?
   (b) Have the parents got unrealistic expectations of the child?
   (c) Are the parents over-concerned about their child's diet, resulting in the child manipulating the parents?
2. Would the child be more successful if seated more comfortably?
3. Is the difficulty caused by poor chewing patterns?
4. Do perceptuo-motor difficulties make cutlery difficult to handle?
5. Is there difficulty in transferring food to the mouth?
6. Does the child need to be taught how to cut food?
7. Could the problem be reduced by a more appropriate choice of cutlery and crockery?

Dressing

Increasing maturity usually results in increasing independence in the activities of personal care. At about 3 years of age children are able to undress and dress provided that they are helped with putting garments on the correct way round. By the age of 4 years most children can dress including fastening buttons. By 5 years they can usually manage all fastenings, including shoe-laces (Illingworth, 1983).

Factors affecting independent dressing

It would be foolish to suggest specific ages at which children accomplish specific dressing skills; as with all areas of development children vary for a number of reasons. In addition to the level of motor and perceptual development, children are given different amounts of opportunity to practise dressing. Parental attitudes towards independent dressing vary. Some are eager for their children to learn to dress independently while others enjoy having dependent children. Some will accept their children's imperfect attempts, others will accept nothing short of perfection. Some children are determined to attain independence at an early age and will struggle to put on garments, refusing help until they are successful. Others have little interest in dressing.

All these points must be taken into consideration when considering dressing. Children may suffer from perceptuo-motor difficulties together with the problems caused by their specific difficulties.

Helping the child with perceptuo-motor difficulties to manage clothes

On occasions when children are being assessed and dressing skills are being discussed parents will apologize for their children's lack of skill, adding that if only they had *allowed* their children to dress themselves there would not be a problem. They plead *mea culpa*. It is important to explain that the fault is not usually theirs. Children will not consistently refuse to dress themselves if they are able to do so. The problem is usually a mixture of the children's perceptuo-motor difficulties and lack of understanding of the problem on the part of their parents.

This is not to suggest that children are never reluctant to dress. There are times when all children are engrossed in an activity which is of much greater interest than dressing. Reluctance to dress may be used as a delaying tactic when it is to be followed by an activity which is unattractive to children. For children with perceptuo-motor difficulties dressing is a complex activity which requires concentration and application. It is also an activity which requires a consistent, methodical approach which is particularly difficult for such children. It is likely, therefore, that they will find more situations than usual when they are reluctant to dress.

There are several basic points which may be suggested to parents to enable them to help develop their children's dressing skills.

1. Do not insist on independent dressing when time is short, for instance on mornings when children must be in school by a particular time. Choose occasions when ample time is available and parent and child can give their full attention to the task.
2. Choose occasions when the child will be highly motivated to attempt dressing. Concentration and application is likely to be focused if dressing is to be followed by an eagerly anticipated activity or event.
3. Minimize distractions such as television programmes and toys.
4. Demonstrate the best position for the child to adopt while putting on a particular garment. This may be sitting on a chair or on the floor, standing or even leaning for support against a wall.

Some types of clothes are easier to take off and put on than others. Begin with garments with which the child is sure to be successful.

1. Garments which are on the large side are easier to manipulate than those which are a close fit.
2. Knitted fabrics have more elasticity than woven ones and are easier to pull on and off.
3. Some children who suffer from perceptuo-motor difficulties have a head circumference which is slightly larger than average. (Sometimes this is a familial tendency and the

head circumference of other members of the family should be noted before it is assumed that a child has an abnormally large head.) Round and polo-necked sweaters and T-shirts which do not have any fastenings at the neck may be uncomfortably tight to pull over the head. For children with perceptuo-motor difficulties, the experience of having a sweater apparently stuck around the forehead, obscuring vision, can be very frightening. The problem may be avoided by ensuring that non-fastening necklines have sufficient elasticity to allow them to pass easily over the head. Alternatively the neckline should have an easily closed fastening which may be opened when the garment is being put on or taken off.

4. A raglan, dolman or batwing sleeve allows more room to manoeuvre the arm down the sleeve than a set in sleeve.
5. Any fastening should be at the front of the garment so that it is possible to visually monitor hand movements while manipulating the fastening.
6. Choose garments with as few fastenings as possible. Some parents may find it difficult to adjust to this suggestion for they enjoy dressing their children in elaborate fashion clothes which often have complicated fastenings, sashes and buttons at the back, buttoned flaps, etc.
7. Traditional school uniform
    Some schools, even at infant level prefer children to be dressed in school uniform.

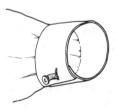

Figure 2.2 A short length of narrow elastic has been sewn to the shirt cuff in the position where the button is usually sewn. The other end of the elastic is sewn to the button thus enlarging the circumference of the cuff and removing the need to unfasten the cuff button when dressing and undressing.

(a) Frequently this includes a shirt with a number of small buttons down the front and at the cuffs. Slim children may be able to take the cuff over their hand without undoing the button. This may not be possible for plumper children. If a short length of elastic is attached to the shirt cuff, the resultant elasticity will allow the hand to pass through the cuff without the need to undo and subsequently fasten the button (Figure 2.2).

(b) Some children with perceptuo-motor difficulties are able to fasten buttons even though they do so slowly. It is particularly important for them that each button is fastened through the correct buttonhole. By beginning to button at the lower edge of a shirt or blouse it will be possible to see if the corresponding button and button hole have been chosen, thus saving the frustration of having to repeat the task because buttons have been mismatched with their holes.

(c) The button at the neck of a shirt is particularly difficult to fasten because the task cannot be monitored visually. In addition, the neck is close-fitting providing little material to hold and the collar and collar band are interfaced which makes them quite stiff. The problem of fastening this difficult button may be removed by sewing the button on to the end of the buttonhole nearest the edge of the garment so that it looks like a conventionally fastened button. A small piece of Velcro should be sewn to the neckband where the button was originally situated and the corresponding piece under the button hole. The neck of the shirt may then be closed by pressing the Velcro together. This method is particularly effective when a tie is worn with the shirt (Figure 2.3).

(d) Tying a tie can also cause difficulties, particularly when it needs to be accomplished quickly, perhaps when dressing after a games or PE lesson. Some children manage by simply slackening the knot and taking it off over the head and replacing in a similar manner. To do this successfully children must be taught how to slacken the knot, in which direction to pull, otherwise the knot may be pulled so tight that it will be impossible to readjust it. Another method of

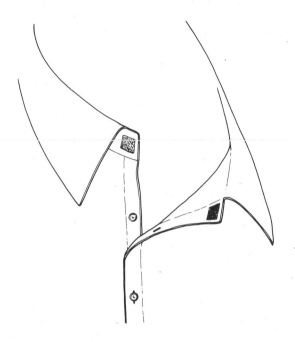

Figure 2.3 The button at the neck of a shirt is usually the most difficult one to fasten. The button and buttonhole fastening has been replaced with Velcro. A small piece has been sewn to the area usually occupied by the button, the corresponding piece has been sewn to the underside of the buttonhole. If the button is then replaced on the outer side of the button-hole, the fastening will be indistinguishable from a normal fastening.

managing a tie is to fasten it permanently and replace the part of the tie which fits round the back of the neck with elastic so that it may be removed and replaced easily. Young children are usually happy with this type of adaptation but older children prefer the former method.

8. Children usually learn to undress before they are able to dress. Some parents need an explanation of this fact. They may also need to be given an inkling of which garments are easiest to put on and those with which their child may experience difficulty. In each case an explanation of the reasons for these difficulties should be given.

9. Most children enjoy dressing up in adult clothes or fancy dress. This interest can be used, by providing appropriate clothing, to improve the children's dressing skills. Children also like to see the results of their efforts in a mirror. This too can be used advantageously to reinforce children's appreciation of their own body image and their body's relationship to the garments.

10. Tying shoe-laces can be a continuing problem for some children. Of course it is possible to wear slip on shoes without any form of fastening or wear those with Velcro fastenings. Unfortunately many of the children who have difficulty with tying shoe-laces also need shoes which provide firm support around the ankle and instep. In some cases only a lace-up shoe will provide this support.

    It is best not to attempt to learn how to tie laces on a shoe which is being worn, for not only will the process of tying need to be learned but also how to position oneself appropriately and reach around one's own knee. It is usually better to begin with something more substantial than a shoe-lace so that it is easy to see the correct position of the knot. A piece of clothes line or rope of similar thickness is suitable. This rope should be tied round a chair rail or other rigid rail or post. Tying a knot should be mastered before any attempt is made to tie a bow. Learning the process by backward chaining, from the end to the beginning, is often effective so that the learner always has the satisfaction of completing the process. For example the teacher demonstrates how one end of the rope is crossed over the other and then the end which is on top is passed down then up through the space formed between the attached rope and the place where the ends cross each other. The learner then pulls the ends until the knot is tight. When the learner can pull in the appropriate direction to tighten the knot the teacher leaves a little more of the process for the learner to complete until the process of tying a knot has been learned.

    Only when knots can be tied with ease should the process of tying a bow be attempted. The preferred method is the two-loop bow. After the rope has been tied in a knot, two loops are made in the ends of the rope nearest to the knot. These loops are then tied together

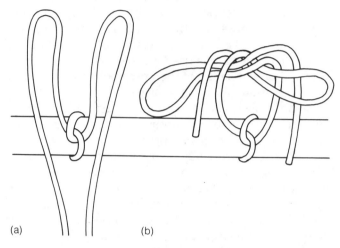

(a)   (b)

Figure 2.4 A two loop bow is often easier to learn than a conventionally tied one. (a) The two loops made after tying the initial knot, (b) Tying the two loops together to form a bow.

by the same process as the knot. The resulting bow will look like a conventionally tied one. The advantage is that the learner will only have needed to learn one basic process (Figure 2.4).

11. There is sometimes a difficulty with putting shoes on the correct feet. Some children with perceptuo-motor difficulties continue to have difficulty appreciating the difference in the shape of the two shoes. (Some manufacturers of shoes such as trainers use the gimmick of printing 'left' and 'right' on the appropriate shoe. This usually does not help because there is frequently a problem with labelling left and right of self and many children are not able to read these two words.) It can sometimes be effective to put an indelible mark on the medial inside edge of a pair of shoes so that when the two marks are apposed to each other the shoes will be aligned correctly with the feet.

PLAY

A large part of the activities of childhood is covered by

the term 'play'. It includes activities involving toys – articles, usually designed by adults, which are felt will be of interest to or of 'educational' value to children. Toys enable children to practise gross and fine motor skills, indulge in imaginative and symbolic play, experience cause and effect, or discover the principles of construction.

Children may engage in solitary play or play together with other children or an adult. Play may involve no additional props, only the child or a group of children. Play may include items found in the home: boxes, chairs and tables, kitchen utensils and clothes.

> All aspects of development, physical, intellectual and emotional, merge in play. The type of play and its role in the child's activities develops with age and maturity but at no stage does it deserve the somewhat derogatory implication in that familiar adult remark: 'He's *just* playing'
>
> Jones, 1973

For most children play develops and becomes more complex as they mature. They develp their own interests in parallel with their motor, cognitive and social skills. It is not usually necessary for parents consciously to guide their children's play from one developmental stage to the next; children usually pursue their own interests in ways which will enhance their skills in all areas of activity.

This is not necessarily the case for children who suffer from perceptuo-motor difficulties. All aspects of play may be affected by their difficulties. Severe difficulties with motor activity are likely to be diagnosed in early infancy. The types of problem associated with perceptuo-motor difficulties are not usually recognized until later because the activities which are affected are not developed until a later age. For example, difficulty with the complex motor planning skill necessary to draw a human figure will not be manifested in the infant, because they have not reached the developmental age when they would attempt such activities. A 3- or 4-year old's attempts at drawing a human figure are usually accepted at whatever standard they are drawn. Unless such a child has undergone expert assessment, motor planning difficulties at this age are often not detected.

In retrospect it may be possible to see that the problems have always been present. It is not usually until precise gross and fine motor skills are expected that perceptuo-motor difficulties may be suspected. Early examples of such difficulties are the child who feels insecure in the bath unless holding on to the sides or handles, the child who paddles a tricycle along with the feet when other children are able to propel themselves with the pedals. (Children can normally pedal a tricycle by the time they are 3 years old; Illingworth and Illingworth, 1984.) Other children with difficulties may prefer the non-specific play of digging in the garden to stacking cubes or nesting cups; they may enjoy watching an adult draw but be reluctant to attempt to do so themselves.

Problems recognized in school-age children

Some children's problems may only be noticed when they have attended school for some time. During the early years, physical education will probably not be structured and children will be free to take part in whichever activities are of interest to them. Children with perceptuo-motor difficulties will probably choose non-specific activities, those which do not require great feats of motor planning or well-developed balancing skills. It may only be when physical education activities become more stuctured that perceptuo-motor difficulties are suspected.

In a similar way, undressing and dressing before and after physical education sessions may initially arouse little suspicion of difficulty because teachers and non-teaching assistants are usually prepared to help very young chldren with the more difficult parts of dressing, such as tying shoe-laces and fastening difficult buttons. It may be considerably later that the child is observed to be much slower and much less adept than most children at removing and putting on clothes.

Many children with perceptuo-motor difficulties manage the elements of lower-case print seemingly without much difficulty. This is particularly true when the child is at the copy writing stage. It is only when more than a few words need to be written that difficulties become apparent. Adding to the problem is the diffculty of performing simultaneous tasks, forming letter characters, recalling the sequence of characters in a word and composing sentences.

Whilst it is not suggested that early intervention would prevent these problems in the school-age child, appreciating their presence and giving the child the opportunity to develop coping strategies would result in less stressful schooldays than are experienced by many children with perceptuo-motor difficulties.

Strategies to help the development of play

It is so easy for a situation to develop where children do not choose to participate in activities which they find difficult, and because they do not practise those activities, they continue to cause problems.

Practise can often be encouraged by breaking an activity down into its separate parts and practising each in isolation. For example a child who has difficulty completing a posting box activity could learn the activity in two parts; deciding which piece will pass through which aperture and having help with aligning the pieces so that they may be successfully posted and secondly learning how to align a particular piece so that it will pass through the appropriate aperture. Approaching a task in this manner will ensure that the child meets with success in each part of the activity and is motivated to attempt the task again until proficiency is achieved.

Many children who have perceptuo-motor difficulties are adept at covering up their problems and diverting adult attention from them. When asked about their child's preferred play, many mothers will comment on an almost obsessional preference for lining up small cars, perhaps taking a favourite doll for a walk in a pram or running aimlessly outside. Whatever the child's preference the activity will usually be one which requires no precise motor or perceptual skill, one in which there is no 'right' or 'wrong'. Appreciating the nature of the child's diversional tactics and the types of activity which are avoided is usually a great help in diagnosing the exact nature of the difficulties.

Gross motor skills and play

The basis of motor skill is body image, appreciating ones own size, height, width and girth, knowing how far one can reach and how small the self can be made by bending and folding the body parts.

It is, however, generally recognized that there is a slowly developing awareness of the infant of himself as separate from his surroundings and that this gradually evolving self-concept becomes for the child a focus point or frame of reference, from which he reaches out to explore the world and orientate himself in space

Francis-Williams, 1970

Many early play and daily living activities reinforce the percept of body image. Bathing and drying the child draws attention to the body parts. They provide tactile and visual input. If these activities are discussed whilst they are taking place there is also auditory input and labelling of body parts. Dressing and undressing, both with regular items of clothing and the play activity of dressing up, provide similar sensory input.

Singing games

There are many singing games which draw attention to body parts and their positions and relationships to each other. Some are suitable for young children:

- This little piggy went to market
- Head, shoulders, knees and toes
- Five little ducks went out one day
- The wheels on the bus

Others can be used to help older children with body image and spatial skills:

- Simon says
- O'Grady says
- Hokey, Cokey

Ball skills

Often the child with perceptuo-motor difficulties is not interested in ball games. Catching, throwing and kicking a ball are complex skills which require good perception of ones own body image, position in space and the relationship of self to the ball and other people participating in the play. They also require concentration and the appreciation of speed and distance.

In order to help the child with such skills, the child's specific areas of difficulty should be appreciated in conjunction with the skills required for the specific activity. It will then be possible to break the skill down into components which the child can practise with a reasonable expectation of success. For example, learning to catch a ball will require the following abilities:

1. Awareness of the position of hands and arms without visual monitoring.
2. Appreciation of the position of the person throwing the ball.
3. The ability to concentrate on the activity.
4. Appreciation of the velocity of the ball and its flight path.
5. The ability to adjust the position rapidly, whilst appreciating the above points, in order to catch the ball.

Thus before being able to catch a ball, the child may need to develop a number of kinesthetic skills.

1. Appreciation of body image.
2. Appreciation of position in space.
3. Appreciation of spatial relationships of self to the person throwing or kicking the ball.
4. Appreciation of the direction, speed of movement and the force muscles exert.

Fine motor skills and play

Many children with perceptuo-motor difficulties will avoid precise fine motor activities. The complexities of jig-saws may be shunned because of problems with interlocking the pieces, perceiving the colour and shape relationships of adjacent pieces or aligning two pieces in the correct orientation to each other. Looking at each part of the activity in isolation will help such a child. The adult working with the child could find the correct piece to fit in a particular position, place it in its correct orientation and then facilitate the child's fitting of the piece, thus providing the child with the satisfaction of completing the process and, hence, motivation to continue with the activity. With another child it may be appropriate to allow the child to search for the correct piece which the adult will fit into the puzzle. Alternatively the adult could select the piece, the child's task being to place it in it's correct orientation before the adult locks the piece into position. Gradually skills are built which enable the child to complete the task without help.

This process may be applied to many activities which will enable the child to build up skills required to complete a task, to be motivated by success to undertake further practice in the activity.

Drawing and painting

Children's interest in drawing and painting activities is variable depending on the opportunities they have to undertake them, the praise and encouragement they receive from peers and parents and the skill they have in manipulating pens, pencils, crayons and brushes.

Many children with perceptuo-motor difficulties will, in the early stages, be happy to apply paint to paper. This is in fact what children do when they are first given paint and brushes, they do not attempt to paint a picture or produce a representation of anything in particular, the task is simply applying colour to the paper. These children may not be so keen to paint when they are expected or feel they are expected to paint a picture. They may have a mental picture of what they would like to represent on paper but are unable to realize it for a number of reasons. They may have difficulty holding the brush effectively or with loading it with paint. They may have difficulty manipulating it to produce the desired strokes on paper or they may not be able to perceive shape or the relationship of shapes to each other.

Similar problems may occur with the use of pencils and crayons. The outcome is often a child who is reluctant to attempt representations on paper by any of the above means. Consequently the child who has difficulties is reluctant to practise and thus there is little improvement in the skill and the sequence of cause and effect, lack of practice and failure is established.

There are a number of elements in helping the child who has difficulty with making representations on paper.

1. Ascertaining the parts of the skill which are causing problems.
2. Working on the elements of the skill which are difficult for the child to accomplish in such a way that the child enjoys success and hence is motivated to further efforts.
3. Using other media for practising strokes in particular directions and accomplishing various shapes:
   (a) strokes and shapes may be carved in wet sand or soil either with a finger or a stick;
   (b) smooth plastic surfaces may be coated with paint and a finger used to remove the paint in strokes or shapes;
   (c) steamy mirrors or ceramic tiles are fun to draw on with a finger
   (d) the grouting between square tiles provides an accommodating groove for small fingers to experience describing a square;
   (e) salt or sand sprinkled on a tray may be drawn upon with a finger or stick.
4. Large stencils (not templates) of geometric shapes can be used to reinforce the proprioception of moving the hand in a circular or other shape (Penso, 1990).
5. Never give the child a complex example to copy, for example a detailed human figure, an ornate house or a car with all technical details. Rather provide the simplest basic example possible so that the child is not deterred from attempting the figure. The child can then add any extra detail which he/she thinks fit and which are within his/her capabilities.
6. Where possible allow the child to copy the movements necessary to complete the shape rather than attempt to copy a completed example. The problem is usually with producing the necessary strokes to produce the shape, not with perception of it; therefore, the child needs to observe and copy the requisite movements.

DIFFICULTIES IN SCHOOL

During the early years of formal education children have

the least personal choice of the activities which they will undertake. Pre-school children are usually allowed to select their own activities within certain limits. Adults on the whole are free to reject activities which do not interest them or which they find difficult. People who have not excelled at sport whilst at school are free to pursue other activities once school days are over. Adults choose occupations and leisure activities to suit their talents. The reverse is true of school children, especially in infant and junior years when there is little or no choice in the activities in which they must take part.

Although children may work in groups, each engaged in a different activity, all children are required to engage in gross and fine motor skills required for handwriting; using scissors, paint brushes and rulers; and performing gymnastics and games. They must learn to listen to instructions and carry them out sequentially; concentrate on activities whilst there is the distraction of the noise and movement of children engaged in other activities in the room. At this stage of life it is, of course, desirable that many activities are attempted. How can talents and interests be developed if a wide variety of activities is not offered?

These early years in school are often extremely difficult for children who suffer from perceptuo-motor difficulties, especially if those difficulties are not appreciated by parents and teachers. Sympathetic handling of such children can make a world of difference from both the children's and the adult's point of view.

When adults understand why children appear to be behaving inappropriately they are able to adjust activities accordingly. Children are presented with appropriate activities and goals and thus success provides motivation for further efforts.

> Clumsy children need understanding, and some need advocates – their difficulties pervade their lives. They come in contact with so many others who may not show tolerance and patience that it is not surprising that, for some, things go wrong.
>
> McKinlay, 1987

Difficulties with handwriting

One of the most precise yet diverse patterns of movement

expected of school children is handwriting. Not only is handwriting expected to be swift and legible but it must be accomplished without conscious effort whilst considering the content and structure of a piece of work, the structure of sentences and the sequence of letter characters within a word, spelling. Children who have fine motor difficulties, problems with motor planning and perhaps additional perceptual problems with orientation and sequence of letter characters will have significant problems with handwriting. The paucity and poor quality of their written output can lead, if their difficulties are not understood, to under-estimation of their abilities.

Schools vary in their philosophies about the teaching of handwriting. Some ensure that children are thoroughly conversant with the correct construction of letter characters before they are allowed to attempt to write words. At the other extreme, some schools allow children to construct letter characters by whatever method they choose, leaving the teaching of their correct construction until a later stage. Between these two extremes are schools which give some guidance about letter character construction, perhaps using completed examples for children to trace over or providing a dot to indicate where to begin forming a characer and an arrow to indicate the direction in which it should be constructed.

Children who suffer from perceptuo-motor difficulties must have precisely structured help in order to realize their potential with regards to handwriting. They will not 'just pick it up'. Areas of difficulty must be assessed and remediation will involve the whole child, not only the hand. Most will need individual instruction to learn correct letter construction. Providing a completed example to copy or trace over is rarely helpful. A kinesthetic approach is often effective, the child learning the necessary movements. A verbal commentary always using the same phrases helps many children.

Sitting position

The overall sitting position of the child affects the resulting handwriting. Schools tend to have only one size of furniture in each classroom. This results in children who are large for their chronological age using furniture which is too small.

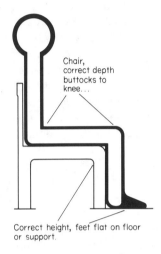

Figure 2.5 Diagrammatic representation of an appropriate sitting position on a chair of the correct size. The depth of the seat comfortably supports the thighs with the knees and ankles at 90 degrees. The chair is of a height which allows the feet to be supported flat on the floor.

Conversely, smaller-than-average children use furniture which is too large, resulting in them balancing precariously with feet unsupported.

Furniture of a size suitable for individual chilren is desirable for all children but vital for those with perceptuo-motor difficulties. The correct size of chair will ensure that the depth of the chair supports the thighs but the front edge of the seat does not press uncomfortably into the back of the knees. The height of the chair will allow the feet to be placed flat on the floor with the ankles and knees at right angles (Figure 2.5).

Provided with the correct size of chair, children with perceptuo-motor difficulties must be taught how to sit on their chairs. They frequently perch on the edge of the seat or sit in a twisted position. Teaching these children to sit with buttocks to the back of the chair seat, with the trunk parallel to the work surface and shoulders in a relaxed position, is vital (Handley, 1986a, 1986b, 1986c; Lewis and Salway, 1989).

The position of paper or other writing surface needs to be given active consideration. Most schools today provide a horizontal writing surface, unlike the past when most children sat at desks which had a sloping surface. There is now once again, a trend towards a sloping writing surface which does indeed enhance the writing position and hence the hand-writing of many children (Wallis-Myers, 1987; Brown and Henderson, 1989). A little experimentation will ascertain if a sloping surface is of help to a particular child and the optimum degree of slope.

The position of the paper in relation to the writer must also be considered and often actively taught to children with perceptuo-motor difficulties.

> In general, the right hander has his paper to the right of his midline and tilted in an anticlockwise direction. The left hander has his paper to the left of midline and tilted in a clockwise direction. The non-writing hand always holds the paper steady.
>
> Alston and Taylor, 1985

Few adults would choose to write on a single sheet of paper placed on a hard surface; most would rest the sheet of paper which is being used on several other sheets or on a large magazine or the like. Similarly, children benefit from having some form of padding between the paper and the surface supporting the paper, particularly if it is of plastic material. This not only makes writing more comfortable but also helps to hold the paper in position. For children who have particular difficulty in preventing their paper from slipping, a thin sheet of Dycem under the paper is often effective.

The importance of attention to these details cannot be overstressed; for position of self, equipment and paper can produce significant improvements in the ease with which children write and the handwriting itself.

Choosing pens, pencils and paper

Just as many school children are provided with a single size and type of furniture at various stages in their education, so many are also provided with one type of writing tool. Children usually have little or no choice in the type of writing point, diameter of barrel or the weight of the tool they use. Children who are provided with a choice of writing tools do not always choose the type that would have most likely have been chosen for them (Jarman, 1984, 1989). Often children are given thick pencils and crayons during their early days in school. Many children would choose, and often handle, a finer pencil or crayon much more effectively.

When helping children with perceptuo-motor difficulties the friction provided by the writing tip should be considered. The more friction provided, the easier the tool will be to control. For example, a ballpoint pen provides very little friction, whereas a felt-tip pen provides a great deal of friction. Such children should experiment with writing tools which have barrels of various diameters until they find the one which is most comfortable. Similarly, various weights of writing tool should be tried. some prefer a heavy tool, especially if the hand has slight unsteadiness. Others find a lightweight tool easier to control. Experimenting with various weights of tool will help the decision of which is most appropriate (Penso, 1990)

Art and craft

Many of the difficulties which are apparent in handwriting also affect drawing, painting and other artwork. Many of the points mentioned above will be relevant to artwork. In particular children with motor planning problems will find drawing frustrating.

Colouring

Colouring a picture with crayons or felt-tip pens will often result in a picture which far from satisfies the creator: colour will extend beyond the outlines and will be applied unevenly. The child with perceptuo-motor difficulties will often need to be taught exactly how to colour a picture. Holding the colouring tool a little higher up the barrel and with a slightly looser grip than when it is used for writing will help the child to make the necessary light and even to and fro movements. When colouring with a pencil crayon, using the side of the lead will create a more uniform effect than using the tip.

Using glue

Craftwork which includes the use of glue will also be difficult.

There are so many elements of the task to consider almost simultaneously. It is essentially a two-handed activity which in itself is difficult. This is accentuated by poor body image, failure to appreciate position in space and spatial relationships of self, between self and materials and between the various materials being used. For some children it may be sufficient to teach very precisely each element in the glueing process. Some children may find a twist up glue stick easier to handle than liquid glue and a brush. Other children with greater perceptuo-motor difficulty may be best, at least for a time, working on tasks where success can be guaranteed. It is not a good idea for children to have the glueing task completed for them. When 'their work' is displayed they are usually very much aware that most of the project is the result of efforts other than their own. This approach does nothing to help self-confidence, self-esteem and motivation which are probably already pretty low.

Case note

Nicholas' fine motor and perceptual difficulties were of such severity that soon after beginning school he began to learn keyboard skills. He also experienced difficulties with drawing, painting and craft work.

His therapist suggested that he should undertake alternative methods of producing art and craft work to other members of his class. His teacher was reluctant to accept this suggestion, feeling that it would make Nicholas feel 'different' from the other members of the class. Most of 'his' work was largely completed by his teacher. He was very much aware that the work was not his own and he became very reluctant to even attempt such activities.

His attitude improved when he undertook his own projects using stencils, printing techniques and arrangements of leaves, flowers and other materials in collages. Although Nicholas was undertaking activities different from other members of his class he felt less 'different' because he was undertaking activities in which he could succeed.

Scissors

Cutting paper and other materials with scissors is frequently a very disappointing activity for many children with perceptuo-motor difficulties. Analysis of the task will prove just how complex it is. It requires the following skills.

1. Perfect hand–eye co-ordination.
2. Rhythmical, reciprocal opening and closing of the scissors to exactly the correct degree.
3. Eye concentration on the line along which the scissors will cut.
4. The manipulation of the scissors must be accomplished without any visual reference to either the scissors or the hand which is manipulating them.
5. The hand which holds the paper must also be adjusted as the cutting progresses so that the paper is continually held in the most appropriate position to ensure smooth progress of the blades of the scissors along the cutting line.
6. In addition overall planning is necessary to plot the sequence in which the shape will be cut out, a difficult task for those with perceptual difficulties.

Many such children will have had little opportunity to develop their scissor skills in pre-school days. They will have had difficulty mastering the skill. Parents may have been reluctant to teach these skills because such children often have poor concentration and perhaps a tendency to wield scissors dangerously near to their eyes and other parts of the body. Because of their awkwardness with scissors many parents decide to err on the side of caution and exclude cutting with scissors from their child's acitvities.

As with other hand skills, the importance of a stable sitting position cannot be stressed too much. It is particularly import-ant for scissor activities where the safety of the child and other children must always be considered.

The choice of scissors is important. Though it may seem obvious, scissors must be sharp enough to cut the material for which they will be used! Yes, scissors can be dangerous but those which are blunt and so encourage the child to use force and yanking of the material can be very dangerous indeed. Blunt scissors, of course, produce very disappointing results for a child who is already having difficulty accomplish-ing a skill.

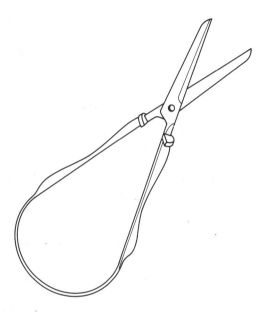

Figure 2.6 Easigrip scissors which require a whole-hand rather than finger movement. The scissors are sprung and therefore open automatically when the grip is released.

Children who hold scissors in their left hand must use left-handed scissors. This ensures that the cutting line is not obscured and that the blades come together as the scissors are closed.

Cutting with scissors requires accurate movement of the index and middle finger and the thumb. Where this movement is not yet adequately developed, whole-hand grip (Easigrip) scissors are usually more appropriate because they completely remove the need for finger movement. They are sprung to open automatically when the grip on them is released and are closed by squeezing them with the whole hand (Figure 2.6).

When holding conventional scissors the thumb should be through one handle and the middle finger through the other, the index finger is placed on top of the handle and helps the middle finger to pull. Using the thumb and middle finger through the scissors handles produces more control and power than using the thumb and index finger. To cut, the hand should be held in a position midway between pronation and supination, the thumb will be in a superior position. Similarly the hand which holds the material to be cut will be held in this mid position with the thumb on top.

Before attempting to cut out anything specific the process of cutting should be taught. For this purpose thin card is more suitable than paper because it is less floppy, easier to hold and cuts more crisply. Offcuts discarded by printers, about 4 cm wide, are ideal for initial cutting practice because the piece of card is severed in one movement of the scissors. The first task should be to snip off tiny pieces. Many children are delighted with this activity, their first success with cutting. When cutting is easily accomplisihed wide lines should be drawn across the strips, a centimetre is not too wide for first attempts. As the child succeeds with cutting within these limits the width of the line is reduced until cutting is successful along a fine line.

The first attempts at cutting out shapes should be of straight-sided figures. Curves require much more control in the adjustment of the direction of cutting with the scissors and adjustment of the position of the paper in the other hand. Because it has the least number of sides, a triangle is the best choice for first attempts at cutting shapes.

It may also be necessary to help children with the order of the cuts made to cut out the shape. Some will attempt to cut an angled shape in one continuous cut which results in inaccurately cut corners as well as difficulty with the paper which is to be discarded. Teach children to consider the lines which will be cut along before beginning the task, then to cut along one line at a time, discarding each section of unwanted paper before a further line is cut. Some children will need to be reminded to begin cutting from the edge of the card or paper.

When these details of the use of scissors are taught children will be successful and that success will provide the motivation for further practice.

3

Do problems disappear with maturity?

A child-like man is not a man whose development has been arrested; on the contrary, he is a man who has given himself a chance of continuing to develop long after most adults have muffled themselves in the coccoon of middle-aged habit and convention.

Aldous Huxley, 1931

There is a range of motor and perceptual competence which is considered to be within normal limits. Those who perform at the highest levels of competency will be considered to be talented in some areas of activity. Amongst this group will be sports people of local, national and international repute as well as those with exceptional practical skills.

The lower limits of what is considered to be 'normal' motor and perceptual ability will vary, depending upon a number of factors.

1. The general expectations of the society within which the person lives.
2. The current age of the person.
3. Attitudes, acceptance and understanding of family and friends.
4. Attitudes towards self.
5. Type of education establishment attended and subjects studied.
6. The type of career which is being pursued and the skills which are necessary in order to be successsful in that career.

THE EXPECTATIONS OF SOCIETY

A primitive society which relies on hunting on foot to obtain an adequate food supply would consider a youth or man who could not run efficiently or aim accurately with a weapon to kill or immobilize the quarry to be abnormal. In a sophisticated society where the supply of meat is dependent on visiting a butcher's shop or supermarket, inability to run swiftly or aim accurately at a moving target does not have the same significance.

Conversely, in a sophisticated society the ability to make legible and swift letter character tracings on paper is considered important. People who suffer from motor planning or visual perceptual difficulties often find that handwriting requires conscious effort and frequently the completed script looks 'immature' and is difficult to read. There may also be problems with lack of speed when writing and even difficulty with sentence construction or spelling. Such difficulties are a significant problem in sophisticated societies. Similar difficulties would probably remain undiscovered in a primitive society where such fine high-level skills would not be significant.

These are two rather extreme examples of the significance of perceptuo-motor difficulties in very different societies. In societies of today the perceptuo-motor competencies which are generally expected vary in a much more subtle way. Within some families and groups, athletic prowess will be highly esteemed, in others fine hand skills will be valued. Thus, even in today's society different perceptuo-motor difficulties will be of greater significance in some groups than in others.

AGE

Motor and perceptual skills develop and are refined as age increases. A child of 2 years does not have the motor or perceptual maturity to be able to write at speed or to cut out complex shapes with scissors. No one would expect to find these skills in a 2-year-old. If a person of 15 years, living in a sophisticated society, has not acquired these skills, that society considers the person, in the absence of discernable physical disability, to be unusual and lacking skills which are considered to be 'normal'.

Physical appearance is also important, particularly in the comparatively young. Generally people expect less of a child who looks younger than his/her chronological years. Conversely the child who is large or looks more mature than the average child of that chronological age will be at a disadvantage, for people will tend to expect behaviour from that child beyond his/her chronological age. Children who are large or mature for chronological age, who also suffer from perceptuo-motor difficulties, are doubly disadvantaged; their skills are probably below average for their chronological age while more is expected of them because they look older than their years.

Particularly during primary school years the child with perceptuo-motor difficulties who is one of the youngest in the class suffers additional disadvantage. For example, in the British education system, children with an August or early September birthday will always be amongst the youngest children in their school year. There will be almost a year's difference between their ages and the oldest children in the class. Perceptuo-motor problems will increase the gap between their abilities and the older children in their school year.

There is a group of children, usually those with mild or moderate difficulties, who at school entry have significant difficulty with perceptual and motor skills whose problems appear to resolve with increasing age. 'Early diagnosis [of clumsiness] need not indicate life-long disability that cannot improve' (Knuckey and Gubbay, 1983). It may be that this group of children who appear 'clumsy' in early years but make significant improvements have suffered from maturational lag; nevertheless, attitudes shown by others and those adopted by self may persist even when perceptuo-motor difficulties cease to cause significant problems.

FAMILY AND FRIENDS

The basis of parental attitudes towards their children is complex. When the first child is born to a family the child is at the beginning of experiencing life; the parents are also new to their role. Their expectations of what that role will be are influenced by their memories of how they were treated as children, advice from family and peers and from media information. Thus expectations of parental role and child behaviour and achievements are extremely variable.

It is understandable that the early signs of perceptuo-motor difficulties are easily dismissed. Some young children are messy eaters, refuse to attempt independent dressing, prefer digging in the garden to activities which involve fine hand skills. Parents can easily rationalize these preferences by such explanations as, their child is always ravenously hungry and therefore eats very quickly, is more interested in play than dressing and prefers outdoor play.

It is often not until the child enters school that it is realized that the child suffers from perceptuo-motor difficulties. The significance which parents attach to perceptuo-motor difficulties in their child will vary from family to family.

1. Some parents will themselves have experienced such difficulties. (This information is sometimes volunteered during assessment procedures, provided parents are encouraged to make their personal contribution to the assessment.) Their attitudes towards their child will depend, in part, upon their own experienecs which may elicit one or more of the following responses.
    (a) 'I understand how s/he feels.' Parents will often describe difficulties very similar to their child's and add anecdotal evidence of personal problems they have experienced.
    (b) 'Nobody helped me and I've managed all right.'
    (c) Feelings of guilt because they suspect that their child has inherited their own difficulties.
2. Some parents deny that their child has a problem. They may assert that their child's problem is one of laziness, perhaps daydreaming or lack of effort. A common plea is, 'He/she can do it if he/she tries.' Yes, it may be true but do such parents appreciate the huge amount of effort their child must put into activities in order to be successful?
3. Some parents will blame their child's difficulties on a particular teacher, teaching methods or lack of facilities in school.

4. Some are convinced that once a particular medical or surgical procedure (often the insertion of grommets in the ears) has been carried out, all will be well.
5. Many parents feel that their child will 'grow out of it' and in some cases they are correct.
6. Some parents will go to great lengths to seek out every possible source of educational and medical help for their child. They believe that they will find a panacea for all their child's problems. Help may be sought from alternative/complementary practitioners in food allergies, acupuncture, etc. Others may seek out educational establishments which have a highly disciplined approach, often concentrating only basic academic subjects. Others will opt for a school which concentrates on personality development rather than academic excellence. There are occasions, of course, when the chosen strategy is highly successful.
7. Many parents will also go to great lengths to prove that their child is of superior intellectual ability. This approach can be justified, for often children who suffer from perceptuo-motor difficulties have difficulty demonstrating, by handwriting and other fine motor means, their knowledge, reasoning, imagination and future potential.
8. Some parents who give great weight to sports and other physical skills will intimate to their child, verbally or by attitude, their disappointment at their child's lack of potential in these areas.

ATTITUDE TOWARDS SELF

How far attitudes towards self are influenced by external circumstances is open to debate. Recent longitudinal studies (Rutter, 1989) have stressed the importance of 'the immediate environment as the main influence on a person's behaviour, ... we should examine the characteristics of the environment that contribute to immediate happiness and well being'. For people with perceptuo-motor difficulties which do not resolve in childhood, the injustices experienced in early years need not lead to continuing feelings of inadequacy, inability and failure. Changing experiences and interactions in the sequence of life can enhance self-esteem and confidence.

Changing life situations can also have the opposite effect. US Air Force recruits who were not diagnosed in childhood as having perceptuo-motor difficulties had their problems highlighted when they were subjected to the military routine of marching, drill and folding bedding (Shelley and Reister, 1972).

Observation suggests that children who have had the reasons for their difficulties sympathetically explained to them, and strategies introduced to overcome or circumvent those difficulties, retain their self-esteem. It is also important to stress to the child his/her value as a person despite any difficulties which may prevail.

Case note

David was referred for occupational therapy because of difficulty with handwriting. Assessment suggested that he had dyspraxia which was evident at both a gross and fine motor level. The nature of his problem was explained to him and his parents, stressing that such problems did not detract from his underlying abilities nor his value as a person.

Treatment concentrated on gross motor skills which were appropriate to age and interest, and basic strategies which would help his handwriting skills.

He is now in his mid teens, has little interest in sport and accepts that handwriting takes more effort for him than for most of his peers. Academically he is making excellent progress.

TYPE OF SCHOOL AND CURRICULUM

At all levels of education, philosophies of learning differ slightly between individual teachers, schools, education authorities. These philosophies will also vary through the years as the result of changes in pedagogic theory and to some extent the needs of industry. In recent years the trend has been away from whole class teaching to learning in small groups. There has been much thought and effort expended on child-centred learning and less time spent in learning by rote.

In particular the swing has been away from handwriting as a desirable skill for its own sake to handwriting being a means of communicating facts and ideas and opinions. Less time is spent, in many schools, learning the mechanics of handwriting and perfecting those skills. Children who suffer from perceptuo-motor difficulties benefit from a highly structured yet child-orientated handwriting programme. At the same time it is to their advantage that the content of written work is considered of greater importance than high quality handwriting.

The various changes of emphasis in education always bring some advantages for pupils with perceptuo-motor difficulties, but also some disadvantages.

EMPLOYMENT

The type of employment in which a person is engaged will be influenced to some extent by past experience and opportunities. Inappropriate types of employment will highlight difficulties. Ideal employment will make use of skills and abilities and those activities which are comparatively poor because of the presence of perceptuo-motor difficulties will not need to be used.

In order for this to happen the person will have had educational experiences where teachers were sympathetic to problems and took a constructive approach to them. Further education and career advice will have been realistic in the light of manifested difficulties. Of great advantage will have been assessment and treatment of a medico-therapeutic nature.

It is also an advantage for the person concerned to understand their own difficulties, their strengths and weaknesses and to appreciate that some tasks will require more time and effort than they do for the average person. Most of all, regarding self as a person of value to society and of esteem within the social group concerned can be of infinite importance in the work place as well as in life in general.

RESEARCH

There are many variables in estimates of how far perceptuo-motor difficulties resolve with increasing maturity, or are helped by remedial programmes, many of which are based on empirical evidence. Valid research into the subject would require large numbers of people who underwent exhaustive assessment as children to be reassessed in their adult years.

In practice, only a small percentge of children who suffer from perceptuo-motor difficulties and adults will take part in such research projects. Inclusion in such a project will, in part, depend on the factors discussed above as well as the severity of the difficulties from which the child suffers. There is also an element of luck: inclusion will depend on the current interest in this subject and the area of the country in which the research is taking place.

Is there evidence that remedial programmes are effective? Evidence of the effectiveness of any programme designed to remediate perceptuo-motor difficulties is fraught with complications. So many questions need to be asked concerning the child, environment, attitudes, expectations, measures of effectiveness, etc.

Children, parents and the home environment

1. Children are immature people who have great developmental potential. It can be difficult to differentiate between skills which have been achieved as the result of a remedial programme and success which follows as the result of maturation.
2. The home environment may either provide children with the space and equipment to foster the development of motor and perceptual skills or lack of such facilities may preclude such practice and experimentation. Some homes are not 'child-orientated' and provide little opportunity for children to experiment and practice gross and fine activities which enhance the development of perceptuo-motor skills.
3. Parental attitudes and expectations can affect children's ability to cope with perceptuo-motor problems and their response to remedial programmes. Some parents persist in denying that their child has a problem and consequently do not make allowances for activities which are difficult for their child to accomplish. For example the child who is reluctant to attempt independent dressing, who has difficulty in recognizing the back and front of garments

and manipulating fastenings may be described as 'lazy', 'awkward' or as 'lacking concentration'. Children who have difficulty with eating may be accused of 'refusing to use a knife and fork' or of 'messing with food'.

Some parents tend to be unrealistic in their expectations of their children. They can be bitterly disappointed when the dainty little girl they imagined their baby would grow into does not materialize. Similarly many boys cause parental disappointment when they do not show what many parents would consider to be 'manly traits' by being the star of the football field or cricket pitch. Children are often very aware of these parental feelings though they remain unvoiced. Their self-esteem suffers and they lack confidence in their ability to succeed even when specific remedial help is offered.

4. The personality of affected chilren can also have a marked effect on the effectiveness of remedial programmes. Some are fired with enthusiasm and resolve to succeed, particularly with activities which are of importance to themselves, while others lack that enthusiasm and tend to give up on activities or components of activities with which they do not meet with immediate success.

Assessments and remedial programmes

1. Perceptuo-motor difficulties have very diverse effects on the lives of sufferers. Signs and symptoms vary greatly between children, both in the severity of a particular symptom and the number of characteristics which are manifested. Remediation will be programmed according to the results of assessment. The remedial programme will therefore be based on the problems which have been noted at assessment. Re-assessment following treatment will be made of the original problems which were observed. Thus, it does not necessarily follow that the *actual* problems have been addressed.

2. Taking into account children's developmental potential, the improvement which is observed may be largely one of maturation rather than any treatment administered.

3. Is attention and sympathetic handling an important element of remediation? Parents often find that spending

time with their child together with a professional who is sympathetic to their problems is extremely helpful. Within a family which includes a child who suffers from perceptuo-motor difficulties, the parents also have problems. They may have difficulty in understanding their child's difficulties and how such difficulties can affect almost every aspect of their child's life. They may find it difficult to explain their child's problem to other people. Sometimes, grandparents, in particular, are loath to acknowledge that their grandchild has a problem. In a school-age child, parents may instinctively feel that their child has considerable ability but because of perceptuo-motor difficulties that ability cannot be demonstrated.

Spending time with a professional who understands these problems, who is able to explain the reason for these problems can often help to dissipate tensions which have built up in the child, in parents, between parents and between parent and child. A relaxed child is more likely to succeed with perceptual and motor skills than one who is stressed and afraid of failure.

Do 'clumsy' children become 'clumsy' adults?

This question is almost as hard to answer as how long is the proverbial piece of string! Today's adults were children 10, 15 or more years ago. Were the assessments of 'clumsiness' as comprehensive as those which would be undertaken today? Were teachers, psychologists, therapists as aware of these problems in children as we are today? How difficult is it to trace people who were the subjects of past studies and are they willing, in adolescence or adulthood, to be reassessed?

Only a relatively small proportion of children who are diagnosed as suffering from perceptuo-motor difficulties, have clumsiness as a sole problem. A percentage also have language and/or articulation difficulties. Others have behaviour, concentration and attention problems. These additional problems may be of greater significance in later life than the perceptuo-motor difficulties diagnosed in childhood. A number of researchers have addressed this question of whether perceptuo-motor difficulties resolve with increasing age.

In 1970 a paper was published by Dare and Gordon describing the assessment, the nature of difficulties and management of 35 children described as having 'a disorder of perception and motor organisation'. 'Most of them had for years been regarded by their parents and teachers as abnormally awkward, clumsy, untidy, difficult and irritating.' The importance of early recognition of the problem, if possible at the beginning of their school careers, is stressed. It is suggested that it is important to give positive advice to the affected child, parents and teachers.

At that time, long-term follow-up of the children in this study or indeed of children in other studies had not been undertaken. These researchers, however, reported that 'there is no doubt that improvement in skilled movements can occur in a relatively short space of time, even in a child of below average intelligence.' This study involved assessment and ensuing treatment; it was designed to be conducted over a comparatively short period of time. We cannot know, therefore, whether the children needed prolonged periods of treatment and support or if the 'improvement' reported was sustained.

Various terms have been used to describe the symptoms of people who have difficulty with perceptual and motor skills. In a retrospective study of 16 young adults at a US Air Force training base, their problems are described as a 'Syndrome of Minimal Brain Damage in Young Adults'. (Shelley and Riester, 1972). These adults, 14 male and 2 female, aged between 18 and 23 years had 'difficulties in learning how to march properly, how to fold and spatially arrange various clothing items and/or Air Force equipment. In general, their speed and ability to learn new motoric tasks (e.g. formation drills, judo techniques, etc.) was felt by the training officers involved to be inferior to those of the other peer group members. ' 'In addition to difficulties in motor performance, these patients had symptoms of marked irritability, anxiety, self-deprecation and emotional lability.' 'All these patients were, initially, grossly anxious and verbalized a concern over their physical and mental abilities.'

None of the subjects' problems had previously been identified. Past history revealed that they had been considered 'sloppy' by their families but had compensated by showing

superior intellectual and verbal skills. Neurological examination revealed no 'hard' signs. 'Soft' signs included 'general
clumsiness', 'poor balance', 'confused laterality', 'disturbed
coordination' and 'poor finger activity' and 'dysdiadochokinesis' in five subjects. On the Weschler Adult Intelligence
Scale the subjects scored between 85 and 124 on the verbal
scale but, predictably, on the performance scale the mean score
was 83.8. The researchers concluded that 'these patients had
avoided areas where a high degree of perceptual or motor competence was required. When they entered the Air force, they
were thrust into a situation which demanded precise, effective visual-motor performance. Careful neurological evaluation and psychological testing indicates that all manifestations
of minimal brain damage do not tend towards spontaneous
remission as has generally been believed.'

Two points in the above study are worthy of note. It
was retrospective; the subjects had not been examined in
childhood and details of their early behaviour is anecdotal.
Their problems had apparently decreased with increasing age
but this was found not to be so when they were in a situation
where they were required quickly to become proficient in the
type of skills which relied on precise motor and perceptual
abilities.

More recently a follow-up study was undertaken of 24 young
adults of between 16 and 20 years of age, 8 years after they
were originally tested and diagnosed as being 'clumsy children'
(Knuckey and Gubbay, 1983). These researchers conclude that
'it is encouraging to learn that clumsiness, as a problem,
is largely confined to childhood itself, rather than a long-
term disability.' '. . .only a small proportion of the clumsy
children are likely to be affected by their disability after
leaving school.' 'This study suggests that for children with
severe degrees of clumsiness there is a less favourable
prognosis. . .'

The study describes how the subjects were retested, after
an 8-year interval, on five of the eight tests of motor proficiency
which were originally used. Four of the five tests were scored
according to the time taken to accomplish them. Speed is not
the only criteria for judging perceptuo-motor proficiency;
though more difficult to measure, quality of movement is far
more significant. It would be interesting to know how these

people fared in real-life situations, when they were under stress, required to perform at speed of undertake unfamiliar motor tasks. Most people endeavour to perform at their optimum level in a test situation when they are able to give their full attention to the task in hand and the environment is free from distractions. Test situations are usually of limited duration, unlike real life where many precise activities need to be undertaken for prolonged periods of time.

One of the most recent studies follows-up, after a period of 10 years, 16 adolescents who were first investigated at the age of 6 years (Losse *et al.*, 1991). The researchers found that 'clumsy' children did not 'grow out' of their clumsiness as has been suggested by other researchers.

> We have shown that the problems associated with clumsiness at age six are still present at the age of 16. This seems true both of academic attainment and for social and emotional adaptation. Moreover, in many instances these increase rather than decrease. Whether there is any direct causal relationship between the motor problems and the other difficulties we observed remains an open question.

These researchers stressed that the tests they administered provided quantitative measures. The results tended to underestimate the qualitative measures. The results tended to underestimate the qualitative differences between the subjects and the control group, as described by their teachers, with regard to handwriting and other subjects which require a high degree of practical skill.

One of the most significant and most disturbing aspects of the study was the incidence of emotional and behavioural problems suffered by the subjects compared with the controls. Many were reported to have poor concentration, were easily distracted, disorganized, forgetful and were under-achieving in school. Some had low self-esteem, were anxious and depressed, had no friends or were bullied and were poor school attenders.

A case study in this report describes a girl who at the age of 5 years had a verbal IQ of 121 and a reading age of 9 years 6 months. At the age of 16 years she was still extremely clumsy and her verbal IQ had fallen to 74. She was reported to being doing badly in school and had low self-esteem.

As more research is undertaken, the long-term effects of perceptuo-motor difficulties of childhood will become clearer. These recent studies are important for they suggest that 'clumsy' children do not necessarily 'grow out' of their difficulties as they mature. Many such children require help and support throughout their educational careers, not only for part of their junior school years as was suggested in the past. The range of skills and the circumstances in which they are employed as school children changes with the passage of years. For example a 6-year-old will be concerned with the construction of letter characters so that small amounts of words may be recorded on paper. A senior school pupil will be required to record on paper legibly and at speed, forming letter characters without giving conscious attention to their construction whilst attending to the content of the piece of work. For people who have perceptuo-motor difficulties the transition from the former to the latter does not necessarily occur without much practice, advice and support.

A number of researchers have commented on the diversity of problems with which the child with perceptuo-motor problems is beset. Many continue to have severe behaviour problems (Gillberg and Gillberg, 1989). Many continue to have a poor physical and social self-concept. There is often lack of confidence, shyness, anxiety, poor concentration, immaturity, aggression and other traits which mar performance and social interaction (Losse *et al.*, 1991). Such problems may prove to be a greater handicap in the long term in the development of a satisfactory lifestyle than perceptual and motor problems. The case studies cited by Anna Losse and her colleagues (Losse *et al.*, 1991) emphasize the serious and continuing problems which are suffered in later years by people who have experienced perceptuo-motor difficulties in their early years.

McKinley (1987) also stresses the continuing needs of children with perceptuo-motor difficulties. 'It may well be that improving the range of general recreational opportunities of young people, with facilitation of access and continuing use by clumsy children, has more to offer the majority than specific individual motor training.' Dr McKinley underlines the point made by Dr Shaffer and his colleagues (1985) that anxiety which is not dealt with in the child who suffers from perceptuo-motor difficulties can lead to 'anxiety/withdrawal breakdown' in adolescence. 'Helping clumsy children is not just a process of physical rehabilitation – it can prevent mental illness in susceptible children and is a process of preparation for adult life.'

Considering all the areas of human occupation and behaviour, recent research indicates that early perceptuo-motor difficulties do not necessarily resolve with maturity. Some people develop their own coping strategies and learn to avoid or circumvent many activities which have previously caused problems. All may be well until unfamiliar and unpractised activities must be attempted, when past problems will again become evident.

Increasingly lack of self-esteem, anxiety and poor peer relationships are proving to be serious and continuing concomitants of perceptuo-motor difficulties. For some people these secondary developments may be more of a handicap than the primary perceptuo-motor ones.

Although adults are unlikely actively to seek treatment for their difficulties many must be aware of their continuing problems, some of which may become apparent when they seek medical treatment for other matters. Many adolescents and adults would welcome the opportunity to learn of coping strategies to help them accomplish activities with which they have difficulties which often cause personal and social embarrassment.

4

Tertiary, further and adult education

With a smile of secret triumph
Seedy old untidy scholar,
Inkstains on his finger-nails,
Cobwebs of his Gladstone collar,

Unaware of other people,
Peace and war and politics,
Down the pavement see him totter
Following his *idee fixe*.

William Plomer, 1950

Formal education which continues beyond the years when school attendance is compulsory may be described as tertiary or further education. That which is recommenced in later years is adult education. Increasing numbers of adults are now undertaking further study, perhaps after a number of years in employment or time spent caring for a family. Some of the latter will previously only have completed the minimum number of years in school, because of lack of opportunity or in some cases because progress during early years in school was frustrated by perceptuo-motor difficulties. These types of education undertaken after the minimum school leaving age may be academic, vocational or undertaken out of personal interest as a leisure pursuit.

People who suffer from perceptuo-motor difficulties will need special guidance with regard both to their capability of successfully completing a course of study and to the suitability of a particular course to lead to further study or employment.

Past experience and performance will provide some indication of a person's strengths and weaknesses and enable realistic advice to be given.

The desire to pursue a particular career often provides powerful motivation to complete a course of study. A student, for instance, who found large amounts of handwriting difficult to complete in earlier years of education may find the prospect of a career in a desired area of work provides sufficient motivation to persevere.

Past performance, therefore, is not the only indicator of future success. The student who is aware of what is involved in the form of written and practical work, both during the course of study and in qualifying examinations, will be well prepared to begin studying. If, in addition, every means possible is taken to minimize the effects of perceptuo-motor problems the student will be helped along the way to success.

Case note

Recently Jane has begun work in her first post as a qualified nursery nurse. Her qualification was obtained as a result of a great deal of determination and hard work on her part and the advocacy of her paediatric consultant and therapists. She suffers from severe perceptuo-motor difficulties.

In secondary school she was fortunate in having a tutor who understood her difficulties, who liaised with her consultant and therapists and included compassionate pastoral care in her duties. Secondary education included a different teacher for each subject on her timetable. Some members of staff were more sympathetic and understanding than others

Handwriting required total concentration and was produced slowly, though the completed work looked neat and was legible (Figure 4.1). At that time IBM ran a scheme whereby reconditioned electric typewriters were sold at a very much reduced price to people with motor disabilities which precluded handwriting or made it difficult to accomplish. Jane used one of these machines but did not become sufficiently proficient to use it to any great extent for school work. Her lack of speed of movement also affected her keyboard skills.

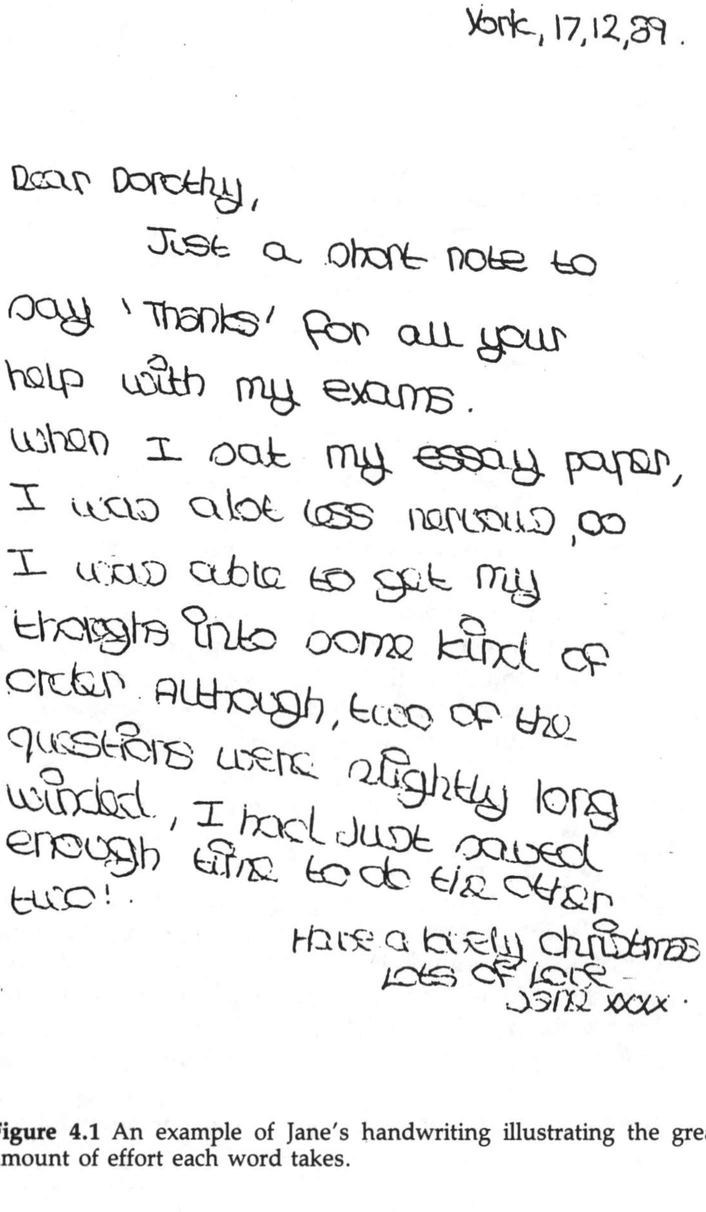

York, 17,12,89.

Dear Dorothy,

Just a short note to say 'Thanks' for all your help with my exams.

When I sat my essay paper, I was alot less nervous, so I was able to get my thoughts into some kind of order. Although, two of the questions were slightly long winded, I had just saved enough time to do the other two!.

Have a lively christmas lots of love - Jane xxxx.

Figure 4.1 An example of Jane's handwriting illustrating the great amount of effort each word takes.

Before sitting her GCSE examinations a statement from her consultant and occupational therapist was submitted to her examination board explaining the nature of her problems and requesting that she should be allowed extra time to complete her written examination papers. With half an hour extra time she attained low average results.

She applied to the local technical college for a place to study to become a nursery nurse. Her application was unsuccessful; she failed her personal interview. It was felt by her year tutor and therapist that this was because her voice is rather monotonous, giving the impression of indifference. There is also a slight delay between being asked a question and her response which could give the impression that she is unable to answer.

Jane was, of course, very disappointed but decided to spend a further year at school studying a pre-vocational course. Before her interview for the nursery nurses course the following year, her occupational therapist wrote to the college staff concerned explaining the nature of her speech difficulties and stressing that her slow and monotonous responses in no way reflected her real ability.

Jane was successful in obtaining a place on the following year's nursery nurses course. Neither the large amount of written nor the project work was easy for her. Some aspects of the practical placements were difficult. She found changing the nappy on a wriggling baby almost impossible. The task became even more difficult when she was required to supervise a lively 2-year-old at the same time! With great resolve she completed the course work.

Before she was due to write her final examination papers her consultant and occupational therapist again requested an extra time allowance. This was refused but after much involved communication with the examination board, they decided to allow her an amanuensis. This concession was made very shortly before the papers were to be written. There was very little time to practice the technique of dictating. Jane failed to gain her diploma by a couple of points. Her self-confidence was rocked again.

Her determination and grit served her well. She returned to her studies, practised planning out the answers to examination questions and the technique to dictating them to an amanuensis. Four months later she gained her diploma. No one deserved her qualification more than Jane; few will have worked harder or with more resolve.

CHOICE OF SUBJECTS

Adolescents and adults usually do not have an unlimited choice in the subjects they may study. As with younger people choice is limited by a number of factors.

1. The range of subjects offered at the educational establishment which they attend. Unless the establishment is very large there will be a limited range of subjects offered.
2. Choice is further limited by the various combinations of subjects it is possible to accommodate in the timetable. For instance, if physics is being taught at the same time as biology, it will not be possible for a student in that year group to study both subjects.
3. Where the choice of subjects studied at advanced level depend on examination success at the previous level, the choice of subjects will be similarly limited.
4. Students who suffer from perceptuo-motor difficulties may have studied a very limited number of subjects to examination standard. Unless they are prepared to spend time gaining further basic qualifications, their choices of courses of further study will be limited.
5. Past educational experience is likely to have some influence on the decisions people with perceptuo-motor difficulties make with regards to further education. Sadly, some will have received little sympathy or realistic help, decide that further education is not for them and leave school at the earliest opportunity.

Choice of subjects to be studied will also depend on the precise nature of the perceptuo-motor difficulty the student experiences. Honest answers to the following questions will provide pointers to the direction further study should take.

1. Am I able to write notes sufficiently quickly to record all the information I will need?

2. Does the course entail writing a large number of lengthy essays? Can I write sufficiently swiftly and legibly for long enough periods of time to complete such essays?
3. Should I consider using alternative means of recording on paper to pen or pencil?
4. Would I be able to record on paper more effectively if I learned keyboard skills in order to use an electronic printer or lap-top microcomputer?
5. Could I or would some other agency fund the purchase of a suitable keyboard?
6. Is there sufficient time to acquire keyboard skills before I begin my course?
7. Can I cope with the practical elements of the course? For example can I handle laboratory equipment, tools or cooking equipment safely?
8. Will I be able to do myself justice in written and practical examinations? Will I need an extra time allowance or other concessions?
9. Is the educational establishment which I propose to attend aware of my difficulties and sympathetic towards them? Do I need a professional advocate, doctor, therapist, psychologist, to explain the nature of my difficulties?

Future career

Subjects to be studied are also chosen because of plans for a particular type of employment in the future. Certain qualifications are needed in order to embark on a particular career. That career will have been chosen after careful consideration of what it entails in terms of both practical, theoretical and social skills. It is particularly important that the person is aware of what the job entails. For example a young person may excel at dealing with clients booking a holiday with a travel firm but perceptual difficulties may make organizing the paper work involved very difficult.

For the person with perceptuo-motor difficulties, compromises may have to be made. The necessary study may include subjects which will prove difficult and require a great deal more effort than for the average student but will be only small elements when in employment. Balanced against the student's past experiences and achievements in formal education are aspirations for the future. Careful assessment of the student's strengths and weaknesses will enable realistic advice to be given which will enable the student to make appropriate choices of study and future career.

Throughout the years of formal education handwriting is frequently an area of difficulty. Many teachers are becoming aware of the problems which arise as a result of handwriting difficulties and are sympathetic to students who experience them. They do not, as in the past, simply advocate practise and more practise as a solution. Extra practise only provides a solution where the problem arises solely from lack of it.

It is particulary important that people who suffer from perceptuo-motor difficulties have adequate teaching of the basic principles of handwriting. They will not just 'pick it up' and need precise, supervised teaching. Dr Rosemary Sassoon has written excellent books about the skill of handwriting (Sassoon, 1983, 1990; Sassoon and Briem; 1984). Where difficulty with handwriting arises from motor planning difficulty (dyspraxia) remediation should be based on demonstration of how the written trace is formed, not on copying completed examples.

There are those with perceptuo-motor difficulties who, despite excellent teaching and adequate practise, fail to develop their handwriting as a realistic means of recording on paper. These are people for whom the precise movements of the writing tool over the paper never becomes automatic. They continue to need to give conscious thought to the ever-changing movements which are required to produce letter characters. They may manage to produce reasonably legible handwriting when they are able to give their full concentration to it. That is, when they are not required to consider, in addition the content of their writing, spelling, sentence construction, recall of information or visual accommodation and figure – background discrimination as when copying from a chalk board or overhead projector. Even without these additional tasks it is unlikely that handwrting will be produced at any great speed. These difficulties should be considered not only with regards to writing examination papers but also as a matter of daily concern with writing sufficiently quickly and legibly to make useful notes and complete essays and projects within reasonable time limits.

Standards of handwriting and the task

Students should realize that different standards and speeds of handwriting are appropriate for different purposes.

1. It is only necessary, for example, for the writer to be able to decipher personal notes for immediate use.
2. Notes which the student will use for revision prior to tests and examinations need to be legible and set out in a manner which facilitates their use as revision material. Because of the length of time involved, it is not usually advisable to rewrite notes. A better strategy is to spend time initially learning the art of making notes, excluding all unnecessary words so that the maximum information is recorded using the minimum of words.
3. Essays and examination papers are written in order to be read by other people so that the script must be legible. An examination script which is legible and pleasing to the eye is often looked upon more favourably by examiners, though this is usually an entirely unintentional response (Briggs, 1980).
4. A great deal of student handwriting is undertaken under pressure, examination papers and essays which will be assessed. This tension and pressure can affect both legibility and neatness (Sassoon, 1990). These points are particularly important for students who also have to contend with perceptuo-motor difficulties.

Subjects and the amount of handwriting involved

More writing, note-taking, essays are required in some subjects than others. Many students will already have discovered this fact and have reached informed or unconscious decisions about the subjects they wish to continue to study.

Generally, the arts entail greater amounts of recording on paper than the sciences. There will, of course, be exceptions to this rule depending on the nature of the course being studied. A course which contains a small or moderate amount of recording on paper will be easier for a person with perceptuo-motor difficulties to follow. The amount of handwriting required to pursue personal interests and aspirations do not always coincide with a person's handwriting ability. How then can students be helped to record on paper the required amount of information with speed, legibility and of pleasing appearance to the reader?

Choice of pen

Handwriting does vary according to the type of pen which is used. By the time the student embarks on further education rules are usually less rigid about the type of pen which may be used. It is not too late to experiment with using different types of pen until one is found which is comfortable to use and produces the most pleasing results.

One which produces a degree of friction is more easily controlled in its trace over the paper. Thus a ballpoint is least easily controlled while a felt or fibre tipped one's friction provides more control. A fountain pen produces pleasing results for some though those who apply a great deal of pressure may not find it effective. Some people with perceptuo-motor difficulties may have problems replacing cartridges of ink without spillages (Penso, 1990).

Appearance of the written page

Beauty may be no more than skin deep yet the appearance of the written page does have an effect on the prospective reader. A neat, legible page encourages its reading. A teacher or examiner who finds the last of 50 or so scripts to be read is untidy and badly presented will be inclined to be less kindly disposed to it than a well presented one. This attitude may be entirely unconscious and not at all intended.

Two projects were undertaken in 1980, the results of which suggest that 'poor' handwriting is marked down where as 'good' handwriting is marked up (Briggs, 1980). Ten essays were each written in ten different handwriting styles. Ten groups of five teachers marked and ranked the essays. The results suggested that handwriting style distorted teachers' perceptions of academic ability. In the second project, five English language scripts were reproduced in five handwriting styles. They were marked by five groups of five teachers. Handwriting style seemed to have a significant influence on the marks awarded. The results of this study are specially significant for examination candidates whose handwriting is impaired by perceptuo-motor difficulties.

Students who have difficulty with the presentation of written work can use some strategies which will make the page appear to be more attractive.

1. Wherever possible paper should have a printed margin so that there is no need for the student to spend time drawing one. This margin should always be respected.
2. Pencils used to draw diagrams, illustrations and graphs should be well sharpened. Drawings using a blunt pencil look untidy. The person with perceptuo-motor difficulties is likely to break the tips of pencils relatively frequently and so will find it useful to have a larger supply of suitably sharpened pencils than other students.
3. Titles and side-headings should always be underlined with a ruler.
4. Where appropriate, a piece of work divided by underlined subheadings will make the page easier to read.
5. Preparing the piece before beginning to write will allow the student to begin new paragraphs appropriately. Each paragraph should be indented discernably and uniformly.
6. Labels for diagrams should be parallel to the top and bottom of the page. Lines connecting the label with the appropriate part should be drawn with a ruler.

Speed of handwriting

Most tests of the speed of handwriting are based on the number of letter characters written per minute. Testing is usually carried out over a short period of time, often between 1 and 3 minutes. A short phrase or sometimes a single word is written repeatedly for the prescribed time (Pickard and Alston, 1985; Taylor, 1987). If the test phrase is practised before the timed test, difficulties with spelling and looking back and forth from copy to writing paper are eliminated.

Such tests obviously do not test the speed of handwriting over an extended piece of work. It is writing for lengthy periods which is relevant to people who are in higher education and it is those who suffer from perceptuo-motor difficulties who very often have difficulty with the speed of prolonged periods of handwriting whilst maintaining legibility.

Some people are able to maintain adequate handwriting speeds for a short time though not for many pages of writing. It is important to ascertain the reason or reasons for this deceleration so that decisions can be made regarding their amelioration and, where appropriate, finding alternative methods of recording on paper.

1. Is there difficulty with motor planning which results in the student needing to give conscious effort to and even to monitor visually the construction of letter characters? It will not be possible to maintain this degree of effort for lengthy periods of time.
2. Is there a motor difficulty such as minimal cerebral palsy in which prolonged precise motor effort causes fatigue?
3. Is the hand disproportionate resulting in a pen grip which causes fatigue? Very long fingers, a short thumb in relation to finger length or a low set thumb can all contribute to an awkward and tense pen hold.
4. Is the problem actually with penmanship? Many people with perceptuo-motor difficulties have associated problems, including difficulty with concentrating on a specific task for prolonged periods, sequencing the content of an essay or answer to an examination question or even constructing complex sentences. Unless the person is observed over a prolonged period any of these difficulties may be perceived as a problem with handwriting.
5. Has the person anything to say? Some people who suffer from perceptuo-motor difficulties also have language difficulties. These may be of a receptive or expressive nature. Such a person may not be skilled in the use of oral language. This often causes problems with written language skills. If it is suspected that a person may suffer from this type of difficulty advice should be taken from a speech and language therapist.

Having ascertained the nature of the difficulty with handwriting and taken appropriate steps to reduce the difficulty as far as possible, it is also necessary to discover the actual speed of handwriting in realistic situations. This will take into account all the types of difficulty mentioned above. To make such a realistic estimate of the speed of recording on paper it is not possible to work in a strictly controlled situation, such as is possible when timing the number of letter characters written when repeating a short phrase or sentence for a prescribed length of time.

It is suggested that realistic estimates can be made if the time taken to write each of a number of essays on a number of different occasions is recorded. If a word count of each essay is made and from this the number of words per minute which have been written can be estimated. An average can then be calculated from the total number of essays which have been timed. It has been estimated that in order to record sufficient information at GCSE 'O' level a student must record between 16 and 20 words per minute (Chasty, 1986).

ANSWERING EXAMINATION QUESTIONS

The piece of work which the student presents may be of the most pleasing appearance but should it not contain the required items of information it will not be well received. The student who has perceptuo-motor difficulties often finds it an impossible task to give sufficient attention to the presentation of work, the legibility of handwriting whilst at the same time giving due consideration to the content of the piece.

Often one of the problems of people who suffer from perceptuo-motor difficulties is that they are unable to organize a task of any kind. Planning a piece of written work is often difficult and requires a conscious resolve to do so. Ideas may abound but ordering them seems an impossible task. Eagerness to begin writing often overwhelms any preliminary thought. It is helpful to be able to demonstrate that a few minutes spent in planning a piece of work can often save time in the long run. In a written examination situation it can also ensure that facts and information are recorded which will gain valuable points.

Work prior to writing the answer to a question should begin with ensuring that the question has been read and understood correctly. Marks will not be gained for information which is not required. Many people who have perceptuo-motor difficulties, find that reading accurately is also a problem. If this is the case, the question should be read several times to ensure accuracy. A personal brain-storming session, writing on scrap paper whatever ideas arise is a good starting point. These ideas can then be rearranged and ordered in the best way to respond to the question.

Such a plan, recording the content of each paragraph in perhaps one or two words will help the student to record only relevant material. The paragraphs can then be numbered in the sequence in which they will be written. This will not necessarily have been the order in which they were originally noted. Time devoted to demonstrating to the student the benefits of preliminary planning to examination papers will be well spent, for not only will the answer be improved but in the long run valuable time will be saved.

Should handwriting be accomplished rather slowly, it is particularly important that the words which are written are meaningful. There should be no superfluous words. The student should be taught how to convey the maximum amount of information whilst writing the minimum number of words. Specific help will often be needed to explain, demonstrate and allow the student to practise such techniques.

Points to stress to the student

1. Read the question and decide exactly what information is required.
2. Note the style of answer which is required; essay, a paragraph or note form.
3. Plan the answer on rough paper using key words.
4. Write as succinctly as possible omitting unnecessary 'padding'.
5. Set out the answer neatly and as legibly as possible.

ALTERNATIVES TO HANDWRITING

There are those for whom recording information by means of

a pen or pencil will never be efficient. Because their problems do not completely inhibit handwriting or are not as obvious to the uninformed as overt physical impairment they may not have been appreciated in the early years of education. This is especially likely to be the case if the student is highly motivated, has determination and has otherwise been a more able student than average. Such students, especially in the past have been regarded as coping adequately. If their handwriting difficulties had been appreciated and accommodated, however, their school performance would have been better than they were able to demonstrate.

Students whose progress is impaired by lack of handwriting speed or legibility should consider alternative methods of recording some or all their work by other means.

Keyboards

It is suggested that learning to use an electric or electronic typewriter or printer or a word processing programme of a microcomputer should be seriously considered. Learning to use any of the above types of machine must include acquiring keyboard skills which will allow maximum speeds to be attained (Penso, 1990).

Students who would like to use a keyboard to complete examination papers should apply to their examination board for permission to do so. Applications should be timed so that there is ample time to clarify specific instructions from their board and make any necessary provision to comply with the board's requirements. It may be that a board will require a particular type of keyboard to be used and if so the student will need time to become accustomed to using an unfamiliar machine.

An appropriate time should be chosen for the learning of these skills and sufficient time must be allowed for skills to be developed before the machine is used for school work. Considering older school pupils, the long break between completing GCSE examinations and beginning 'A' level studies is a good time to acquire keyboard skills.

OTHER STRATEGIES FOR COMPLETING EXAMINATION PAPERS

Sometimes simpler means will suffice to allow students to

demonstrate their skills and knowledge in written examinations. An extra time allowance may be all that is necessary. Some students will take full advantage of every minute of extra time. Others may actually use very little of it but will be able to approach the examination much more calmly and confidently knowing that extra time is available should they need it. The amount of extra time allowed is at the discretion of examination boards and may vary according to the nature of the disability from which the student suffers.

It is important to apply to the examination board concerned in good time. For examination papers which will be written in May or June, application should be made at the beginning of the year. Enquiries should be made regarding the best time to apply for an extra time allowance. Usually the application needs to be supported by a statement from a doctor or a therapist who knows the applicant stating the nature of the problem which makes an extra time allowance necessary. It is also helpful if an estimate is made of the percentage of extra time which will be required, based on the applicant's speed of handwriting in a realistic situation.

Some examination boards suggest that the examinee should have an amanuensis should there be difficulties with handwriting. On occasions, some boards have preferred a student to complete a paper in this way rather than giving an extra time allowance. Dictating to a scribe will be a new activity for most students and time will be needed for practise so that the student and scribe feel comfortable with the procedure. Dictating is a skill not usually practised by students and requires information to be organized mentally before it is verbalized. Writing to dictation may also require practise unless the amanuensis is used to the task.

PRACTICAL SUBJECTS

Handwriting is not the only skill which may impede the progress of the student who suffers from perceptuo-motor difficulties. The manual skills required in laboratory work, design and technology, home economics and handicrafts may also give rise to problems. Some of these difficulties may not have been so apparent in earlier years because students often work in pairs or groups, so that the inability of one pupil will not necessarily be obvious in the finished piece of work.

It may be possible to adapt some work so that it may be accomplished by the student with perceptuo-motor difficulties. For example, some chemistry equipment could be held with clamps secured to a firm base so that fewer items are hand held. Full attention can then be given to the equipment which it is necessary to manipulate.

Cooking equipment may be secured with Dycem mats and the use of a food processor safely taught so that the need to chop, slice or grate food by hand is eliminated. Some students will need individual instruction before they feel comfortable and competent with some techniques.

Similarly, the use of a sewing machine which has the capacity to complete many functions automatically will enable the student to produce precise buttonholes, blind hemming, etc. Generally time spent in becoming proficient in the use of a sewing machine will be more profitable than time spent practising hand sewing. The latter requires precise, regular, rhythmic movements which are often difficult for people with perceptuo-motor difficulties to attain and sustain.

Care should be taken to ensure that special provision is not being made to enable the student to undertake course work where it would be unrealistic for the student to undertake such activities in the course of future employment where special facilities would not be available. However, some courses contain projects which do not need to be undertaken again in subsequent employment. This emphasizes the need to ensure that the qualification to which the course leads will be one that provides opportunities for exploitation of the realistic abilities and skills of the student but will not entail activities which will give rise to undue difficulty.

ORGANIZATION OF SELF

Perceptuo-motor difficulties do not only affect the accomplishment or motor and perceptual skills *per se* but also of general organization of self. These difficulties may include confusion with time, sequence and space.

For the student, time is valuable and its use must be planned to maximum effect. Help may be needed when planning projects so that an appropriate amount of time and effort is given to each part. Students may need constant reminders of time they must allow for library and practical research. It is so easy to daydream rather than write, particularly if a piece of work has not been adequately planned. The need to plan pieces of written work, the topics it will contain and the sequence of those topics cannot be over-emphasized. It is a skill which may have to be deliberately taught and frequently revised.

Plans will also be required when revision prior to examinations is being undertaken. Notes or texts may be 'read' and 'reread' without their content being noted. A fluorescent marker pen may be helpful in drawing the eye to key words. Listing key words on each topic may help others, particularly if they are numbered so that the student knows the number of key facts to be recalled within a topic.

METHODS OF WORKING

Working in short bursts of high concentration is usually more effective than longer periods of less highly motivated work. A timed half hour of work followed by 10 or 15 minutes of an activity unrelated to the subject being studied, in a different room, will result in more work being accomplished than during a long continuous work period.

An overall plan of revision in preparation for examinations will also be needed so that the whole syllabus can be adequately covered. Books are available for each examination subject which set out the syllabus in a logical order and suggest realistic strategies for revision. The support of a friend or mentor may be helpful in ensuring that the proposed plan is realistic and that it is being followed.

Students should also ascertain their best method for remembering facts. Some most easily commit to memory visually presented material, others have a more effective auditory memory. Some remember best kinesthetically, in this case by writing and rewriting material.

The effect of the emotions on memory should not be underestimated. Working with a fellow student, revising together, seeing the humorous side of course work can all help with committing course work to memory.

5

Personal appearance and the impression given to others

In clothes as well as speech, the man of sense
Will shun all these extremes that give offense,
Dress unaffectedly, and, without haste,
Follow the changes in the current taste.

Moliere, 1661

'Appearances are deceptive' we are told. In the case of the person with perceptuo-motor difficulties this may be all too true; the impression they give to the world in general may be very different from the 'real' person within. Posture, gait, gesture, clothing and the effects of personal grooming may all give an erroneous impression of the personality and characteristics of the person concerned. 'Beauty is only skin deep' and 'beauty is in the eye of the beholder' are sayings familiar to everyone; nevertheless, we *are* impressed by personal appearance and demeanour. Help which can be given to people with persistant perceptuo-motor difficulties in order to make the most of their appearance will be beneficial not only in the world of work but also in everyday casual and continuing relationships with others. 'He ought to look neat and tidy. It's half the battle ... making a good first impression,' wrote J.B. Priestly (1946).

That appearance is important is illustrated by the increasing amount of evidence from interviewing. 'Research shows the interviewer's first impression is made after only 30 seconds and a final decision takes four minutes' (Sheard, 1991). The same writer comments, 'An interview often has little to do with reality. It's about impressions rather than facts. Research shows that 55 per cent of an interviewer's decision depends on the candidates grooming'.

The impression transmitted to others does not depend, in the main, on being a 'trendy' dresser, having an up-to-the-minute hairstyle or the application of complicated cosmetic techniques. Such techniques do have some effect on others but overall posture, gait, facial and body gesture override superficial effects.

POSTURE AND GESTURE

The basis of good posture is appreciation of one's own body image and position in space and spatial relationships. 'The development of body image is a continuous process from birth throughout life to death.' Body image 'is the awareness of the body including knowledge of body parts and their relationship to each other and laterality, i.e. the internal awareness of the left and right sides' (Ogilvie, 1978). Only when a person has a good appreciation of body image is it possible to appreciate one's own position in space and relationship to other objects in the environment (Penso, 1987).

Some people who suffer from perceptuo-motor difficulties will not be aware of these concepts and their relationship to posture and graceful movement. Many such people who are adults today will not have had the benefit of therapeutic intervention during the years of childhood. An explanation of these principles, without the use of professional jargon, will often provide an insight into the basis of the difficulties and a starting point for self-help of the person who suffers from such difficulties. It will be possible to consider the configuration of the body parts, their relationship to each other, how far the body may be extended and how small a space it may occupy when all the joints are flexed. Consideration of length of reach with the arm, length of stride and the space the feet occupy will help to make conscious movement more graceful. It is debatable whether or not appreciation of body image and spatial concepts can become completely unconscious or automatic in the person with perceptuo-motor difficulties.

Physical activities

Very often people with perceptuo-motor difficulties are not interested in physical activity of any kind. In particular, they are not drawn to team games which involve contact and swift reaction to the actions of other team members. For many such people, physical activity of any kind often does not have any great attraction.

Attempts to interest such people in individual activities will usually meet with more success than encouragement to take part in team games. Suggestions of trying golf, darts, archery, swimming, water sports such as canoeing, or exercise systems where speed is not of the essence, are more likely to be successful because there is no need to react swiftly and accurately to the actions of other people. There is time to consider position in space, the body's relationship to equipment, to plan movements before they are carried out, to consider distance and the amount of power which must be exerted by muscles.

The exercise system known as Callanetics (Pinckney, 1989) may be attractive because the movements are simple; there are no complex sequences of movement to master. Each exercise concentrates on very small movements of a single muscle group and each participant works at her/his own level of competency and speed.

Finding some form of physical activity which such people find interesting is important for a number of reasons, not the least of which is the reinforcement of appreciation of body image and spatial concepts and hence posture. The trunk muscles are often poorly developed which can encourage poor posture in standing as well as sitting. Small adjustments of the trunk muscles play a large part in overall balance; muscles with tone are better able to fulfil this function than lax, poorly-developed ones. Any activity which increases the tone of the trunk muscles will be beneficial.

Very few people have a perfectly symmetrical body; those with perceptuo-motor problems may have more asymmetry than the average person. In some instances this is the result of a very slight motor deficit on one side of the body. Activities which include bilateral movement such as rowing, canoeing or swimming will help appreciation of equal power and range of movement on each side of the body. The resulting direction of movement, whilst swimming for instance, will make it obvious if one side of the body is working more power-fully than the other. Such activities will also reinforce a sense of rhythm and the grading of movement.

'All or none' responses

Grading of responses and actions can be a major problem, particularly in social situations. There may be difficulty with voice modulation, appreciating the loudness and pitch of the speaking voice and grading volume in all the shades between a whisper and a shout. The speaker may be unaware of the voice problem but aware of the reaction of others towards them. The advice of a speech and language therapist will be valuable once, of course, the speaker is aware of the problem.

This same response may also contribute to affective responses such as laughing and weeping. Some people have difficulty grading their reactions to emotive situations in that they either do not show any amusement at all or are convulsed with laughter. Similarly, weeping may be of an all or none nature. Whether or not this problem can be remediated is debatable. It may be that if such people are made aware of their unusual reactions they would be more able to temper their responses to become within the norms of their social circle.

CLOTHING

Why do some people look great in almost anything they wear yet others seem never to 'get it quite right'? For people with perceptuo-motor peroblems this problem of choosing appro-priate clothes and wearing them effectively can be a real difficulty affecting self-confidence in many life situations. There are a number of basic points to consider which will help to enhance the flattering aspects of clothing.

1. The choice of garments to suit the figure.
2. The colour of garments to suit the colouring of the complexion.
3. The garments which are combined to make an outfit.

4. The suitability of the garment for the occasion on which it is being worn.

These are considerations which everyone must make when choosing which garments to buy and selecting them from the wardrobe each morning. Some people seem to have a natural flair when choosing clothes, others gradually learn from experience, reading articles and books on the subject and the advice of friends.

Adults who suffer from perceptuo-motor difficulties may not develop these skills automatically as their experience increases. They may also have additional problems in combining garments to make an outfit and in the general appearance they present.

Helping adults to choose clothes

Garments hang better on a person with good posture. Many people who suffer from perceptuo-motor difficulties find maintaining an erect symmetrical posture difficult. It is possible to improve posture by exercise though it is doubtful if strategies which are learned will become automatic and integrated into everyday posture. Clothes therefore should be chosen, as far as possible, so as not to emphasize poor posture.

A well cut set in sleeve with, where appropriate, a small shoulder pad will give a neater appearance to the shoulder line than a raglan or unpadded dolman sleeve. Bell-shaped sleeves which are wide at the wrist should perhaps be reserved for special occasion wear. Inaccurate perception of one's own position in space and relationship to other objects can make movement hazardous, particularly in unfamiliar surroundings or when undertaking unfamiliar activities. The addition of an uncontrollable piece of material dangling from the arm can increase those hazards. Reaching across the dining table can pick up a variety of foods and sauces in such errant folds of fabric! Other activities such as washing dishes can be equally hazardous.

Trousers which have a non-slip inner surface to the waist band will hold a shirt or blouse in place more securely than one made of slippery lining material. A shirt or blouse made of matt surfaced material will not pull out of a waistband as easily as one made of shiny material. Some men still choose to wear nylon shirts, often because they need little ironing; unfortunately, this is the type of material which slips out of a waistband most easily. For both men and women a neatly fitting belt will help to keep a shirt or blouse in place within a trouser or skirt waistband.

Some people who suffer from perceptuo-motor difficulties do not automatically sit elegantly. This problem will be particularly obvious when wearing a close-fitting, straight skirt, especially if it is short. An easy-fitting skirt with fullness will make this problem less obvious.

Choice of fabrics

1. Wherever possible fabrics should be washable, preferably by machine. People with perceptuo-motor difficulties are particularly prone to let drips from cups, morsels of food, drops of soapy water when washing the hands, etc., fall on clothing. Easily washable clothing enables a smart appearance to be more easily maintained.
2. A pattern printed on or woven into fabrics can enhance their serviceability. Plain fabrics with a plain weave tend to show even the slightest mark. Very pale colours and black show up marks particularly easily. Pattern, especially if it is multicoloured, and texture in the form of fancy weaves or irregular spinning of yarns, tend to make soiling less obvious.
3. Fabrics which are formed of yarns which are loosely meshed together, such as some fancy tweeds and tricot fabrics are easily stretched out of shape. Such fabrics can quickly become unsightly: trousers become baggy at the knees and narrow skirts become baggy around the buttock and thigh area.

Choosing flattering clothes

1. Most of us have had the experience of being told that a particular colour is especially becoming. We feel good wearing some colours whilst other shades seem to do nothing to enhance the appearance. Particular colours complement certain skin and hair tones. This is equally

true for men as for women, though some men have reservations about accepting this.

Skin tends to have golden, pink or bluish undertones, each with hair and eyes in any of a number of shades. Choosing clothes in colours which enhance these basic skin tones lights up the face and flatters the skin. Carole Jackson (1980) in her book, *Colour Me Beautiful*, explains in detail how to arrive at the range of colours which will be most flattering.

2. Having a wardrobe of garments in a coordinated range of colours will not only flatter the skin tone but will also make co-ordinated outfits easier to select. For example, if greys and blacks form the basis of the wardrobe other clear colours such as turquoise and royal blue, deep pinks and purples will blend with them. Should the most flattering basic colours be in the brown range they will blend with other shades in that group such as terra cotta, golds, yellow-greens and orange shades.

3. In recent years, buying a coordinated outfit has become much easier since shops and department stores have begun to display coordinating garments together. This makes shopping easier for people who have difficulty choosing garments which are suitable to be worn together. For some people dressing will be simplified by wearing these co-ordinated garments together and not attempting to mix and match within the whole range of garments in their wardrobe.

4. Wearing garments appropriate to the occasion is also important. A bikini is appropriate on the beach but would attract stares if worn in a city street. Overalls are appropriate apparel for repairing a car but would not be so appropriate for a dinner engagement. These are, of course, extreme examples to illustrate the importance of wearing clothes appropriate to the occasion.

Before decisions can be made about an appropriate wardrobe of clothes, lifestyle must be considered. What type of clothing will be appropriate for work, for leisure time and formal wear? Usually the larger part of the wardrobe will be worn at work, unless a uniform is worn. Even if this is the case it may be necessary to choose items suitable for wearing underneath a uniform. The first consideration should be, is this garment suitable to wear for work? Will it combine well with other garments in the work wardrobe?

5. Very few people have a perfectly proportioned figure. Legs may be too long or too short in relation to the length of the body. Bodies may be long or short-waisted, top-heavy or pear-shaped. Careful choice of garments with regards to the cut, shape and length can go a long way towards disguising figure faults. This is particularly important for people who suffer from perceptuo-motor difficulties who have problems of posture, movement and rhythm to contend with in addition to any physical imperfections they may have.

Footwear

Many of the points discussed above regarding clothes also apply to footwear. It should, of course, be coordinated with the outfit being worn and both should be appropriate to the occasion. There are other points to consider which apply particularly to people with perceptuo-motor difficulties.

1. Fashions in footwear change, especially for women. No shoe can look elegant if it impedes gait and the rhythm of walking. Perceptuo-motor difficulties can impair balance which makes high, slim heels difficult to walk in. The balance of the shoe can also affect balance of the body. High-heeled shoes which are constructed so that the base of the heel is in line with the centre of balance of the body encourage a good balanced gait. On the whole, the narrower the base of the heels the more difficult it is to balance on them.

2. The thickness of the sole of shoes can affect ease and confidence when walking. For many people with perceptuo-motor difficulties a relatively flexible sole through which the wearer has some sensation of the surface beneath the feet makes for more confident walking.

3. For people who have a tendency to trip, thick soles which have a welt are not advisable. Firstly because it is easy to trip over the welt outstanding at the front of the shoe. Secondly the wearer may step on the welt

at the medial side of the shoe on the supporting foot, again causing the wearer to trip.

4. It is best for everyone if they wear well-fitting shoes which are snug round the heel while allowing the toes sufficient room for movement. For people who suffer from perceptuo-motor difficulties it is particularly important that shoes fit well round the heel and do not allow the foot to slip forward. Many such people easily invert or evert the foot if the shoe does not hold it firmly, particularly when walking on a slightly cambered or uneven surface. It is also important that the toes are not cramped, for there is often an abnormal reflex which causes the toes to claw the sole of the shoe when balance reactions are activated. This clawing of the toes can also occur when attempting to maintain loosely fitting shoes on the feet.

5. The heels of some women's shoes have a slippery type of plastic on the walking surface which can skid on wet or icy surfaces. It is best if such shoes are re-heeled with rubber or leather before wearing out of doors. New shoes with very shiny soles can also be hazardous. Gently sand-papering the soles before they are worn will reduce slipperiness. Shoe soles with very matt surfaces can be equally hazardous because they will not glide at all over some surfaces and may cause the wearer to trip. This problem is not easy to remedy so it is perhaps best not to purchase such shoes.

Clearly many of these criteria are most easily met with laced shoes or those with a high front. It is easier to find shoes which fulfil these criteria for men than women. In recent years, however, fashionable shoes for women which are also supportive have been easier to find.

Spectacles

It is important that spectacles fit well. The supplying optician will usually be happy to re-tighten any screws which loosen with prolonged wear. Spectacles which slip down the nose can be irritating to the wearer and do not enhance the appearance. The optician should be able to remedy the problem by a slight adjustment to the ear-piece and thus the length of the arm of the spectacles.

Umbrellas

For most people an umbrella is the most convenient item to carry as protection from a sudden shower of rain. It is often held so as to face oncoming wind for maximum protection. Usually there is no difficulty adjusting its position suitably according to any change in direction of wind, or when the user turns to walk in a different direction.

Such manoeuvres are often difficult for people who suffer from perceptuo-motor difficulties, particularly if the user is walking along a crowded street and possibly talking to a companion at the same time. This combination of walking, talking, adjusting the direction of walking to avoid bumping into other people and manoeuvring an umbrella may all require conscious consideration and prove impossible to undertake simultaneously. An impermeable raincoat is likely to be a more realistic solution to protection from the rain.

MAKE-UP

Many women choose to wear make-up everyday, others use it in the evening or for special occasions. Some women feel better able to face the world wearing make-up; they do not feel dressed without it. Make-up may be used to enhance the appearance of the face, to follow a current fashion, to disguise blemishes or as a form of decoration. For whatever reasons a woman chooses to wear make-up to be effective it must be skillfully applied. The various cosmetics must be applied accurately, uniformly and smoothly blended.

Many of the skills which must be employed to apply cosmetics effectively are difficult for the women with perceptuo-motor difficulties to attain. The skill required for the methodical application of foundation with systematic blending, the accurate placement of lip colour and eyeliner and the placement of blusher in order to enhance the face do not develop automatically for many women with these difficulties. A number of techniques can be suggested, however, which will help to produce a more effective make-up.

Foundation

All types of foundation will be applied more evenly and

smoothly to skin which has been prepared. Foundation will cling to flakes of skin and any areas of dryness. Before applying foundation the skin should be cleansed with soap and water, a cleanser which is used with water, or a cleansing cream or lotion. The application of a moisturizing cream or lotion, according to skin type, will provide a smooth base over which the foundation will glide. Moisturizer should be applied sparingly or the foundation will slip! It is best to wait a few minutes between application of moisturizer and of foundation.

The choice of foundation will depend on skin type, personal preference and the prevailing fashion. Some prefer simply to apply a slightly tinted moisturizer to give a smoother effect to the skin, others prefer a foundation with more opacity which will cover minor skin blemishes.

Opinions vary regarding the shade of foundation which should be used. To some extent shade is dictated by fashion, the shades of other cosmetics being used and the desired completed effect. Remember the pale faces of the sixties with false eyelashes and heavy eyeliners; compare them with the more natural effects produced with present day cosmetics.

It is easier to achieve a pleasing effect with foundation if a shade as near as possible to the skin tone is chosen. Such a shade will be easier to blend along the jaw line so that the transition from the foundation on the face and the natural unmade-up tone of the skin of the neck will be imperceptible. The choice of shade should be made in natural light. Colours are distorted in artificial light, particularly fluorescent types. It is best to test shades by applying a small amount to the face along the jawline. The skin on the wrist or back of the hand is not the same colour as the face, therefore they are not good areas for testing the suitability of shades of foundation.

Generally, the heavier the foundation the more difficult it will be to achieve a natural effect. Heavy foundation is not kind to older skin because it will emphasize enlarged pores and the like. In addition, it is difficult to apply evenly. It is best to develop a sequence in which the foundation is always applied so that all areas of the face are treated. So as not to have a heavy application at the jawline and forehead it is best to begin in the middle of the face and work outwards.

It is essential that all cosmetics are applied in a good light, especially so for people with perceptuo-motor difficulties. A mirror on a stand which can be held in one hand and moved as necessary to see the face from various angles is also useful.

Eye make-up

These are perhaps the most difficult items of make-up to apply. Again the items used, the types, the methods of application and the colours chosen will in part depend on the prevailing fashion. No attempt is made to suggest any particular fashion effects but to make general suggestions about techniques which will enable the person with perceptuo-motor difficulties to achieve pleasing effects.

It is easier to apply subtle shades of eye shadow than the more strident ones. Soft shades – taupe, brown, and maroon are more effective and easier to blend than blues, greens and other harder, more definite shades. Matt shades are easier to apply effectively than opalescent ones; the former are also more flattering if the skin of the eyelid is slightly crepey. The areas to which eye shadows and highlighters are applied will depend on eye shape and size, whether the eyes are close or wide set, protrude or are deep set and, of course, current fashion.

Eyeshadow and highlighters can be applied more easily if the application of foundation has included the eye area. It is best to apply colour sparingly; it is easier to apply a little more to achieve the desired effect than to remove part of an over-generous application; the latter often results in it being necessary to begin the whole process again.

Mascara can be particularly difficult for people with perceptuo-motor difficulties to apply.

Case note

Jane, a 20-year old woman, has had help from an occupational therapist since the age of 4 years for her perceptuo-motor difficulties. At the age of 15 years she became interested in using make-up but had great difficulty in applying it effectively. This was partly due to the unsteadiness of her hands and partly to her inability to grade the pressure she used when applying cosmetics.

Sadly, Jane's mother had died when she was 9 years old. She often recounts how her mother had said to her, 'Promise me, Jane, that you will never use mascara because I am sure you will poke your eye out if you do!'

Today, Jane uses mascara and a whole range of other cosmetics effectively. With practice and experimentation with methods of application and mirror positions no one could discern from her completed make-up the problems from which she suffers.

A mascara wand with firm, spirally set bristles will aid smooth application, avoiding lumps of mascara clogging the eyelashes together. Mascaras which have filaments to make the lashes look thicker are more difficult to apply evenly than those without filaments.

A hand mirror or one on a stand whose position is adjustable, will facilitate the application of mascara. The position of the mirror should be adjusted to be in line with the direction in which the mascara will be applied. When applying to the under surfaces of the upper lashes it is helpful to have the mirror above the level of the eyes and look up into it. Conversely, when applying to the upper surface of the lower lashes the mirror should be below the level of the eyes. It is helpful to steady the elbow or forearm on a firm surface and, maybe, the hand on the side of the face.

Initially the aim should be to apply mascara to the tips of the lashes working with smooth gentle strokes. Mascara has most effect on the tips of the lashes and attempts to work too closely to the roots of the lashes could result in macara being applied to the edge of the eyelid. As with all cosmetics it is better to apply a little which can be added to than over-apply which may necessitate removing the make-up and beginning again.

Blusher

It is more effective to add colour to the face by means of blusher than by using a darker shade of foundation. Again fashion will dictate the exact shade of blusher which is used and how it is positioned on the face.

Blushers are available in either powder or cream form. Many people find powders easier to apply than creams though choice is a matter of personal taste and the effect which is desired. Usually it is advised that it should not be applied nearer the centre of the face than the middle of the cheek bones and that applying it in an upward and outward direction is most flattering. Generally lighter shades are easier to apply and blend than darker ones. A large soft brush with a short handle is the most effective way for most people to apply blusher.

Lipstick

The precise application of lipstick enhances the mouth and can be used to hide minor imperfections. Many people who suffer from perceptuo-motor difficulties experience similar problems when applying it as when applying mascara. Similar strategies can be employed to enable effective application. A mirror held in an appropriate position and the arm steadied on a firm surface will both be helpful.

A new lipstick with a finely shaped tip may be quite effectively applied directly from the stick. Once the fine tip has worn away it is better to apply the lipstick with a brush. It should have soft short bristles which provide a blunt not a pointed tip. The added avantages of applying lipstick with a brush are that the colour can be worked well into the skin so that it is longer lasting and that the film of colour will be smoother and thinner than that applied directly from the stick.

CARE OF THE HAIR

Hair is perhaps the feature which it is most easy to alter, both in style and colour. The shape into which the hair is dressed can greatly enhance or detract from the appearance. Time devoted to discussing a suitable style with a sympathetic hairdresser or helpful friend will be well spent.

The foundation of any hairstyle does not rely on how the hair is dressed or on the application of styling preparations, but on a good cut. For those who find styling techniques difficult, a good cut will make the procedure noticably simpler. When suitable, a permanent wave which can be washed and finger dried will eliminate the need for complicated styling techniques.

Washing and styling hair

A spray attachment which fits onto the wash basin taps or a

hand held shower will facilitate thorough wetting and rinsing. Unless thermostatically-controlled, special care must be taken to ensure that the water is of a comfortable temperature before beginning to wet the hair. Some people will find it easier to wash the hair whilst bending over the bath because it provides a larger area into which the water may drain and there is less likelihood of water spilling on to the floor.

Before beginning to wash the hair it is wise to collect together and place within easy reach all the items which will be needed – shampoo, conditioner and towels. Today, most containers of hair-care preparations are of plastic or other unbreakable materials. Any glass containers are best avoided because they are so easy to drop when grasped with wet hands. Plastic containers are very light especially when almost empty and so are easily knocked over when reaching for them when vision is obscured by hair or water. It is worthwhile finding containers which have a dispenser, nozzle or inner cap with only a small hole so the containers which are tipped over will not spill their entire contents. Such a device will also help to grade the amount of liquid which is dispensed from the container.

Some modern hair styles, if well cut, can be left to dry naturally. Other styles will require the use of a hair dryer and brush, heated tongs or hot brush. People with perceptuo-motor difficulties may have initial problems with managing this equipment. The problem may be complicated by the necessity of monitoring the procedure in a mirror and having to appreciate that the movements as seen through the mirror are in fact mirror images of the movements made. Practise may not make perfect though persistent practise will certainly improve skill. Some hairdressers are pleased to help clients improve their home-styling techniques. They will explain that good results rely on styling the hair into a good shape and concentrating on the direction in which the hair should lie in the completed style rather than working on curls, waves and the position of small sections of hair except in the final stages of styling.

EATING IN PUBLIC

People who have had eating difficulties during childhood often retain remnants of them during adult life. Such problems may not cause great difficulty when eating at home but can cause embarrassment when eating in public. A number of simple strategies may help in such situations.

1. Sit with the chair well drawn in to the dining table. Sit straight to the table with the body parallel to the edge of the table and the feet flat on the floor. This will provide a well balanced position and minimize the distance food has to be transported between plate and mouth.
2. Use the serviette provided to spread on the lap and thus prevent fragments of food and drips of liquid soiling the clothes.
3. Choose items from the menu which are easy to eat! Foods such as spareribs and corn on the cob which are usually hand held are difficult to manage. A conventional flat round *pizza* will be easier to cut than a folded and puffed *calzoni*. Similarly, a slice or fillet of meat will be easier to cut than that which needs to be cut away from a bone.
4. Learning to manipulate long pasta such as *spaghetti* or *tagliatelle* is best left for home practise.
5. Ensure that tumblers and wine glasses are not over-filled.
6. Ask for items on the table to be passed. Do not reach for them, lest other items are knocked over on an often small and crowded restaurant table.
7. Give the cutting of food full concentration. Use the knife to gently cut the food; do not attempt to pull it into pieces which can so easily result in food skidding off the plate on to the table.
8. Do not be tempted to take over-large pieces of food into the mouth. They are hard to hold on the fork as well as being difficult to chew and move around the mouth.

LEFT-HANDEDNESS

Estimates of the incidence of left-handedness vary according to the tests which are used to ascertain hand preference, though recent studies suggest that it is about 10% of the population. (Enstrom, 1962; Clark, 1970; Lyle and Johnson, 1976). Dr Clark (1970) found, like other researchers, that in the sample of primary school age children there was a larger proportion of boys (10.9%) than girls (6.5%) who were regarded as being left-handed.

Left-handedness itself usually does not give rise to any difficulties, though a percentage of left-handed people may be described as pathologically left-handed. If a person is left-handed for pathological reasons, poor performance in the non-preferred hand, the right, would be expected. This would include the group of people who suffer from perceptuo-motor difficulties.

> Pathological left-handedness is not confined to groups with obvious signs of brain damage but can occur in more subtle forms in cases where there is no hemiplegia or hard neurological sign.
>
> Bishop, 1990

There is likely to be a higher proportion of pathological left-handed people than right-handed people. Approximately 90% of the population is innately right-handed and 10% left-handed. If, hypothetically, 10% of this whole population have a neurological impairment which causes shift of handedness, 9 people will become pathologically left-handed but only one will become pathologically right-handed. Thus, some manifestly left-handed people will have no neurological difficulty but others will. During her extensive studies of handedness, Dr Bishop (1990) has calculated that 'just over one third of left handers with very poor non-preferred hand skills are pathological left-handers.'

It seems reasonable to postulate that a proportion of these pathologically left-handed people who suffer from subtle forms of neurological deficit will be people who could also be described as suffering from perceptuo-motor difficulties. If allied difficulties such as difficulty with differentiating between left and right of self and of others, difficulty with making sense of mirror images and directional skills are taken into account, pathological left-handedness greatly increases difficulties.

People who inherit left-handedness and in whom there is no pathological causation or perceptual difficulties usually have no problems in adapting to life in a largely right-handed world. Those who suffer from perceptuo-motor difficulties in addition to being pathologically left-handed will find coping with the skills of daily life difficult, and their actions will appear to be particularly clumsy.

Articles and equipment designed for a right-handed world

1. Many irons have the flex connected at the right side of the handle which suits right-handed people but trails over the surface being ironed when used by a left-handed person. Irons are available where the flex is connected to the top of the iron which is equally suitable for use in either hand.

2. Public telephone systems are arranged to suit right-handed people.

3. The thread on screws is arranged so that when tightened with a screw driver held in the left hand the user is screwing towards the body, a weaker movement than working away from the body.

4. Tumblers and cups are usually placed at the right-hand side of a place setting, which is inconvenient for a left-handed person.

5. Saucepans and other receptacles with a handle have the pouring lip positioned to be used when held in the right hand.

6. Hand-operated tin openers are constructed to suit right-handed people.

7. Left-handed people need scissors constructed, in both the handles and the blades, to suit their handedness.

8. Writing a cheque and its counterfoil stub requires a left-handed person to perform cross-handed contortions, particularly when the last few cheques in the book are being written and a wad of used stubs need to be held down. Some banks have substituted pages at the front of cheque books where details of cheques written are recorded. This is an easier system for left-handed people to use but leaves on view to observers previous cheque details.

9. Back-fastening bras have hooks on the back right which can be difficult for left-handed women to manipulate.

10. Side-fastening skirts have zips and hooks on the left, an arrangement designed for right-handed people.

11. Purses with a twist fastener are arranged to be opened with the right hand.

So many devices are arranged to suit the majority of right-handed people. People with perceptuo-motor difficulties who are also pathologically left-handed often find coping with very ordinary situations in daily life full of problems which need conscious consideration. Any advice or treatment they are offered should take into account these additional difficulties.

GAG REFLEX

Everyone has a normal gag reflex which is activated when the pharynx is touched. It is a safety mechanism which prevents food being inhaled. Some people have a particularly sensitive gag reflex so that they gag when the back of the mouth is touched by something other than masticated food. This sensitivity can cause problems in a number of situations.

Brushing the teeth

Some people gag when the molars are being brushed, particularly their medial and posterior surfaces. Gagging occurs most readily when the neck is extended, flexing the neck reduces the tendency to gag. Therefore gagging can be reduced if the back teeth are brushed with the head bent forwards with the neck flexed. Some people like to monitor their teeth brushing in a mirror. This can still be done with the neck flexed to prevent gagging if the mirror rests on a horizontal surface rather than the more usual vertical one.

Effective cleaning of the teeth depends upon applying sufficient brushing movements to all surfaces of the teeth. This in turn depends upon the person brushing her/his teeth having the necessary manual dexterity to sustain the gentle reciprocal of brushing at the same time as moving the toothbrush in order to reach every surface of each tooth.

Dysdiadochokinesis, difficulty with rapid reciprocal movements, is a symptom which can impair effective movement of the toothbrush. Spatial difficulties can impair ability to manipulate the toothbrush to reach all surfaces of the teeth. The combination of small rapid reciprocal movements of the brush combined with systematically moving the brush over the surfaces of the teeth can be difficult. Such problems can, over a period of years, lead to poor oral hygiene. A toothbrush with a small head may make it easier to reach all surfaces of the teeth as well as being less likely to cause gagging when applied to the teeth at the back of the mouth. People who experience such difficulties can be helped by using disclosing tablets after brushing the teeth. These will stain areas of remaining plaque, indicating areas of the teeth which require further attention.

An electric toothbrush may be helpful, for the user need only concentrate on applying the brush to all surfaces of the teeth, the reciprocal brushing movements being undertaken by the vibration of the brush. Some electric toothbrushes are fuelled by batteries housed in the handle of the brush. They increase the weight of the brush considerably and also mean that the handle is of quite a large diameter. For some people this type of electric toothbrush will not be comfortable to use.

Dental treatment

Treatment usually takes place today with the patient in a reclined or semi-reclined position. This does not usually cause problems when the dentist is working on teeth near the front of the mouth, but difficulties with gagging may arise when the back teeth are being treated. It may be difficult to tolerate alginate-filled plates, particularly if the alginate oozes beyond the posterior edge of the plate, when they are being used for taking impressions for crowns and dentures.

Most dentists are sympathetic to gagging problems but they can only be so if they are made aware of them. Gagging can be reduced when impressions are being taken if a more upright posture is adopted, of course, with the approval of the dentist concerned. Most dentists will suggest to their patients that they breathe through their nose while the plate is in their mouth waiting for the alginate to set. It helps if the pattern of breathing quite slowly and deeply is established before the plate is inserted in the mouth and sustained until it is removed.

SWALLOWING TABLETS

Swallowing tablets is difficult for some people. In some instances the problem can be solved by requesting medical preparations in other forms, usually as a liquid.

Some medications are only available in tablet form. This is often because the drug needs to be released slowly. Such tablets are usually very close textured; obviously they must be swallowed whole if their slow-release characteristic is to be retained. The prescribing doctor or dispensing pharmacist will be able to advise if tablets must be swallowed intact.

Tablets are manufactured in many different sizes and shapes. Similarly the size of the gullet differs between individuals resulting in greater ease or difficulty with which tablets may be swallowed. Should the tablet be ovoid or torpedo shaped, it should of course be placed on the tongue so that it passes down the throat along its narrower sides, i.e. it should be placed on the tongue with its longer sides parallel with the sides of the tongue. This is an obvious point but often not considered by people who have become anxious regarding their ability to swallow tablets.

Coordination of the abilities required to swallow tablets is often impaired in people who suffer from perceptuo-motor difficulties. Memories of past failure to swallow tablets, of perhaps choking whilst trying to do so, causes apprehension when it becomes necessary to repeat the process.

No attempt should be made to swallow the tablet with only one gulp of water or other liquid. The tablet should be placed towards the back of the tongue though not so far back that it evokes the gag reflex. The tumbler or cup should contain sufficient liquid for a number of swallows. A number of successive gulps should be taken, concentrating on swallowing the liquid rather than the tablet. The tablet will usually be swallowed with the third or fourth gulp of liquid.

USING SPINHALERS

Many people have difficulty taking medication by means of a spinhaler. The coordinated effort of inhaling whilst activating the spinhaler with the hand can be difficult. Spinhalers are now available which do not require this coordination of hand movement and breathing; the device is first set in its activated position so that the drug will be released when it is placed in the mouth whilst inhalation takes place. Research has been undertaken on some models to ensure that the stated dose is delivered.

BLOWING THE NOSE

Blowing the nose effectively requires the coordination of holding the handkerchief over the nose, inspiring, closing the mouth so that when exhaling no air escapes through it and exhaling. People who have difficulty with this skill often have not considered the elements involved in the task and so are not clear about the skills involved.

An explanation of the elements of the task will help more effective execution.

1. Hold the handkerchief or tissue over the nose, firmly but without compressing the nostrils.
2. Breathe in and hold the breath in.
3. Ensure that the mouth is closed so that when breathing out, no air escapes through it.
4. Breathe out, quite forcibly through the nose so that any mucus is expelled.
5. Carefully wipe the nose clean.

It may be necessary to practise each element separately and gradually put the elements together until the complete skill is learned.

STANDING ON PUBLIC TRANSPORT

Many people who suffer from perceptuo-motor difficulties have problems with balance and saving reactions. Trunk control may be poor and therefore not used to its optimum extent in situations where balancing skills need to be employed.

Travelling on public transport, buses and trains, does not always make for the smoothest of journeys, particularly if the passenger is standing. Passengers will be able to balance more effectively, should the vehicle stop or start erratically, if they stand with the feet comfortably apart so that they are standing on a broader base. Balance will be further aided by standing with the knees slightly bent in a relaxed position and using adjustment of the trunk muscles as an aid to balance.

CONSTIPATION

Many parents of children who suffer from cerebral palsy describe the problems their child has with constipation. It is possible that this problem could be partly caused by poor coordination skills; difficulty with contracting the abdominal muscles and at the same time pushing.

People with perceptuo-motor difficulties may have similar coordination problems, though to a less severe degree. In addition such people may undertake little physical exercise because of poor ability. Exercise is well known to aid the passage of food through the alimentary canal. People who have chewing difficulties often choose a diet which lacks fibre which again can lead to a tendency to constipation.

Unless the constipation becomes severe people are unlikely to seek professional advice about it. Professionals who come into contact with such people should be alert to the possibility of perceptuo-motor difficulties being a strong element in the cause of the problem.

6

Career choices and difficulties

When little Dickie Swope's a man,
He's go' to be a Sailor;
An' little Hamey Tincher, he's
A-go' to be a Tailor:
Bud Mitchell, He's a-go' to be
A stylish Carriage-Maker;
An' when *I* grow a grea'-big man,
I'm go' to be a Baker!

James Whitcomb Riley, 1899

There are very many factors which influence the career people pursue, not all of which arise directly from conscious decisions of the people concerned. The pervading economic climate at the time of seeking the first employment situation will influence the number of posts and type of work which is available. In economically difficult times firms will not be in a position to make big investments in apprenticeships. The number of employees may be reduced through redundancy and natural wastage. Firms will look for value for money in the applicants who are accepted for employment.

Recent years have seen the development of new types of work and some traditional jobs have disappeared as the result of technological advances. The political climate and educational philosophies will influence the ways in which training for work may be obtained and the number of people who will be accepted onto courses. In short, there are many factors which affect career choices in addition to personal inclination and abilities.

Choices are also influenced, particularly in the case of young people, by family and friends. A girl or boy may consciously choose to follow in the footsteps of a parent or relative. Equally, they may decide that the last career they would like to pursue would be one similar to that of a parent! Some young people are greatly influenced by their peer group and endeavour to obtain a post which has prestige in the eyes of that group. Immediate financial gain can often be the prime consideration for many young people and this consideration may blind the person to the possibility of career advancement, job security or the opportunity to gain experience which could be useful in future job applications.

The range of career choices can become limited long before an individual begins to consider the reality of future employment. Fairly early in secondary school career, subject options have to be decided. Most adolescents have some personal choice in these decisions. Teachers will influence some of these choices according to their perception of the ability level of the adolescent. It may be decided that a pupil of low average ability would fair better attempting to study only one foreign language rather than two or three. A general science course may be considered more suitable for some children than studying chemistry, physics and biology as separate subjects and in more depth.

Children may themselves, perhaps unconsciously, make subject choices. A clash of personalities between child and teacher may result in the child rejecting a subject. Conversely, a teacher who motivates and has a good rapport with a child may encourage that child to pursue, with enthusiasm, a course for which there is not a great deal of innate ability.

Organizing a school timetable which accommodates the subject choices of a large number of children is no easy task. Often there are 'casualties', it being impossible to fulfil every choice of every child.

Case note

During his third year at secondary school, Paul was required to decide which subjects he wished to study to GCSE level. Very much a scientific, rather than an arts orientated person, he asked to study mathematics, chemistry, physics and biology. Because of difficulties with the school timetable, physics and biology lessons were taught at the same time so it was not possible for pupils to study both subjects.

At that time he was told that he would be able to resume biology for 'A' level study. This proved not to be the case, thus reducing his career opportunities at the age of 14 years.

The choice of career of all young people is influenced by, at least, some of the factors described above. For those who, in addition, suffer from some configuration of perceptuo-motor difficulties the choice may be even more limited and decisive factors may be evident even earlier in life.

We have seen in earlier chapters how difficulties with fine motor skills, particularly with handwriting, can lead to a child being under-estimated in school. Such attitudes towards a child sometimes develop in the infant department and more often in the juniors. Clearly it is important that all children with such problems receive sympathetic consideration and realistic help from the earliest age.

There are teachers who appreciate the nature of these problems and realize that large amounts of practise with fine motor skills is unlikely to completely resolve the difficulty. In most instances, modifications need to be made in the quantity and quality of fine motor output expected of the child. For some children the method of recording on paper may need to be different from that used by other members of the class. For example, keyboard skills may be used to record longer pieces of work and those which will be displayed in the classroom. Providing a child with alternative means of recording on paper, even if it proves to be a temporary measure can prevent a child's abilities from being under-estimated and in the long run can have a beneficial effect on eventual career choice.

It is vital, therefore, that if a therapist finds on assessment that a child has neurological problems which are likely to impede fine motor skills, that this information is given to the child's school. The nature of the problem and the effects they are likely to have should be clearly explained in non-medical terms to the child's teachers and parents. Teachers also need to know exactly how the child may be helped and activities which are likely to cause particular problems. Teaching staff change and children transfer to different schools. Therapists should ensure that every teacher who handles the child is aware of the problems.

In Chapter 1, the characteristics which often occur together with perceptuo-motor difficulties were mentioned (Henderson and Hall, 1982). There is often speech delay and social difficulties which affect relationships with peers and mentors. Such children often have low self-esteem, lack self-confidence; frequent failure to reach expected goals can lead to lowering of motivation and self-expectations. How can such children, despite adequate intellectual ability, be expected to aim for a high rung on the career ladder?

Early experiences do affect the transition from school to beginning a career in paid employment. 'The point that comes over most strongly from longitudinal studies, however, is that the outcome of transitions, and the ways in which they are dealt with, is partially determined by people's past behaviour and experiences' (Rutter, 1989).

SCHOOL SUBJECTS AND FUTURE CAREER

For the person with perceptuo-motor difficulties there is further conflict between requirements of school and those of a career. There are subjects or areas of subjects which must be mastered in order to gain qualifications for a particular type of employment which will not be used once in employment. For example, English and mathematics are prerequisites of beginning most further education courses. Many students with perceptuo-motor difficulties have a specific difficulty with numerical skills. Others find the large amounts of written work required in an English course extremely difficult to complete. In the world of work, few are required to complete extensive pieces of hand-writing or to solve mathematical problems *per se*. Many people with perceptuo-motor difficulties need an influential advocate to plead their cause during this transition from school to the world of work or further education.

CONCOMITANTS OF PERCEPTUO-MOTOR DIFFICULTIES

Recent research has illustrated that the other problems which frequently occur with actual perceptuo-motor difficulties can have highly significant effects on the life of the affected person (Losse *et al.*, 1991). This was a follow-up study of 16-year-olds who had been assessed as having perceptuo-motor difficulties 10 years previously. Not only were certain skills formally reassessed, but consideration was also given to how they were coping in school, with their peers and with life in general. Many of the emotional and behavioural problems which are reported to occur in these young people will most certainly affect their decisions about whether to continue to further education and their choice of employment.

Lack of concentration is reported by teachers together with lack of self-confidence and anxiety. These characteristics could be constitutional though it seems likely that they are the result of specific difficulties with the gross and fine motor skills in school. They are highly significant when these young people enter the job market.

Another important skill when in employment is the ability to associate with colleagues and communicate with superiors. There were a number of reports in the above study of subjects who were shy, had no friends, had difficulty forming relationships or who were bullied or picked on. If such people are to become successful in employment during their adult years these behavioural problems will need to be addressed as well as the perceptuo-motor difficulties. These behavioural problems could be a severe impediment to retaining paid employment.

COMPLETING APPLICATION FORMS

Applications for places on college and university courses, as well as positions in paid employment usually require the completion of a printed form. Sometimes it is stated that the application should be made in the applicant's own hand-writing. On other occasions the choice is between completing the application form with a typewriter or word processor, and hand-writing it. For the person with perceptuo-motor difficulties there could be difficulty with both methods of completing the form. Yet the application form is often the first contact the applicant has with a prospective employer or selector of students for academic courses. Primary selection may be made from the application forms received. Choice will depend on the qualifications of the applicant and information submitted on the form. The selector may also be influenced by the appearance of the form; the extent to which this is so may depend on the type of vacancies which are to be filled. The manner in which a form is completed can, therefore, be crucial to the result of the application.

Whichever method is chosen to complete the form, it is important first to make a rough copy of the information which will be inserted in each section of it. The vocabulary to be used, the construction of sentences and the sequence of information can then be formulated before beginning to work on the form. In this way it is also possible to ascertain how many words will fit into each section of the form and thus calculate spacing appropriately. People who have particular difficulty in completing forms may find it helpful to make two or three photocopies of it. These can be used for practise before completing the original form which will be submitted.

If the form is to be completed in handwriting the strategies described above will allow the applicant to concentrate on handwriting rather than content when completing the copy of the form which will be submitted.

It can be extremely difficult to adjust the spacing of a typewriter so that the type is appropriately positioned within the allotted spaces. Practice with photocopies of the form may help but cannot ensure exact positioning on the 'real' form. This kind of spacing, which requires a variety of spacing judgements to be made will be particularly difficult for the person with perceptuo-motor difficulties. A solution to this difficulty is to use a word processor rather than a typewriter. The editing facilities of the programme will allow the spacing to be pre-determined and trial runs, which will be identical with the submitted version, to be made. If the copies are made on lightweight, translucent paper it will be possible to place the completed copy over the original and see if the printing coincides with the spaces on the form. This may be time-consuming, but it is worthwhile on occasions where it is essential to submit a form which is pleasing to the eye.

INTERVIEWS

Most people are a little daunted and, indeed, nervous when

they are required to attend an interview. The suggestions which are given to everyone faced with such an occasion are particularly relevant to people with perceptuo-motor difficulties.

Preparation

1. Have as much knowledge as possible about the firm or educational establishment to which the application has been made. This will enable questions to be answered in the light of the needs of the firm and pertinent questions to be asked in addition to the applicant showing a real interest in being appointed to the post.
2. Be prepared to give reasons why that position or educational place is being sought. This is not the time to be over-modest, but neither must the applicant appear to be over-confident.
3. Be prepared to describe one's own suitability and qualifications for the post or place.
4. Interviewees are often asked if they have any questions they would like to ask. Have one or two questions ready.
5. Practising interview techniques in role play exercises and the like with a teacher, therapist or career adviser can be helpful. It is all too easy for the applicant to imagine that they have prepared mentally for the interview only to find that in a real interview situation they are lost for words. Trial runs cannot, of course, anticipate how the actual interview will proceed but can provide some insight into the atmosphere of the situation and the appropriateness of responses.
6. Decide which clothes will be suitable to wear at the interview. Ensure that they are clean and well-pressed. Brand new clothes are not usually the best choice, particularly for people who have difficulty with posture and body image. If necessary practice wearing the clothes before the day of the interview to make sure that they feel comfortable and part of self. If necessary seek advice about the types of clothes in which it is appropriate to attend an interview.
7. Comfortable shoes are particularly important for those who have an awkward gait. Shoes with a wide heavy welt are

not advised because of the danger of tripping. For women, shoes with a very high narrow heel are not usually appropriate for wearing at interviews. They are particularly unsuitable for women with an awkward gait, posture or balance difficulties because they tend to throw the body out of balance and accentuate such problems.

8. Plan travelling so as to arrive in good time. Some interviews take place within a large campus or complex of buildings so that it is important to allow time for seeking directions to, and reaching, the interview room.

9. The tension of the event can lead to the applicant adopting a very tense sitting position. Practice before the event, if necessary, with a therapist or constructively sympathetic friend to advise.

WHICH COURSE WILL BE MOST SUITABLE?

People who are moving directly from school into further education are often influenced in the choice of continuing study by subjects which they have found interesting and enjoyable at school. Some will give little thought to the eventual employment to which that course of study may lead. Others, perhaps of more practical mind, will look upon further education as a means to achieving the first step on the ladder of a desired career.

People with perceptuo-motor difficulties must give serious consideration to both these steps. They must ensure, as far as is possible, that they will find a course of further education interesting and hence motivating. Also, the employment to which it leads must be realistic in the light of the type of perceptuo-motor difficulties from which the person suffers.

They should ascertain the amount of written and practical work the course contains and the pace at which they will be expected to progress. They should be aware of the types and numbers of new skills they will be expected to acquire during the course. This knowledge should be used when choosing a course of study but it should also be tempered by the personality of the student. A highly motivated student with resolve and perseverence will be prepared to devote the many extra hours which may be necessary to complete course work satisfactorily. The knowledge that a course will lead to a coveted career will spur many students to exert the necessary extra effort. An example of a highly motivated student is described in Chapter 4, pp. 66–68. Another case now follows.

Case note

Anna is a student who has shown extraordinary resolve in her efforts to realize her ambition – to be a teacher of history. Before realizing her ambition, Anna will have to record an extremely large number of words on paper, perhaps the largest number of words which are required in any academic subject. The main area in which she has difficulty is handwriting.

For both her GCSE and 'A' level examination papers, her occupational therapist's request for extra time allowances was granted. Anna was very thankful for this extra time, without which she would not have been able to complete her papers. The extra time was most appreciated in the first set of shorter examination papers. At 'A' level, however, where 3-hour papers are set, 25% extra time allows the student to continue writing for the best part of 4 hours. Sustaining the precise motor planning and motor output of handwriting for this length of time is nigh-on impossible for a person with problems in this area. Anna did not gain a sufficiently high grade in her history papers to take up the offer of a place at her chosen university.

At present she intends to retake the examination next year, postponing the beginning of her university course. She has the necessary resolve and motivation to succeed. How can she be assured with any degree of certainty that her fine motor deficit will not prevent success in next year's examinations? Should it be suggested to her that she undertakes a course of study which requires less hand-writing? Is she aiming for unrealistic, unattainable goals?

Elements of a course of study which should be considered

1. How much handwriting will be required?
    (a) Will the course include a large number of formal lectures from which students will be required to make

their own notes? The legibility of handwriting will need to be considered when writing at speed if the notes are to be usable for revision. It is not usually considered a good idea to rewrite notes because of the large amount of time involved. This is particularly true for people who have handwriting difficulties who will already spend more time completing written work than the average student.

(b) Will the course require a large number of lengthy essays or written projects to be submitted? Will the speed and legibility of handwriting make this a feasible possibility?

2. Will typewritten work be acceptable? If so has the student already got keyboard skills? Will it be possible for the student to obtain a suitable machine?

3. Would some other device be more suitable for note-taking, such as a microwriter or microscribe?

4. Another necessary skill will be the ability to extract from lectures pertinent information which must be recorded. This is a separate skill from actual handwriting and many people with perceptuo-motor difficulties will not develop this skill automatically but will need to consciously learn it.

5. Will the course necessitate drawing technical or geometric figures, graphs or other types of illustrations? Does the student have the necessary motor skills to produce these? It may be possible to use microcomputer programmes to produce graphs and some technical and geometric drawings.

6. Does the course contain a large element of practical work? Often students who have had difficulty in school with academic subjects which require large amounts of handwriting are attracted to further education courses which contain a large practical element. In school, pupils often work in pairs or groups and the difficulties experienced by a pupil who has perceptuo-motor difficulties may have been hidden by a partner or other members of the group undertaking most of the work. Does the prospective student really have the necessary precise motor and perceptual skills necessary to undertake practical elements of a course?

7. Will the student be assessed mainly on course work or on examination papers written at the end of the course? Continuous assessment of course work, while requiring

the student to maintain a sufficiently high standard throughout the course, removes the stress of preparation for a single period of examinations and, of course, the need to write examination papers swiftly, legibly and at length.

8. Will the course include work placements? Taking into consideration the behavioural difficulties which may occur, together with motor and perceptual ones, will the student be able to manage social contact satisfactorily?

The characteristics of perceptuo-motor difficulty and its concomitants should be measured against the requirements of the course. Though the skills that will be required after a course has been successfully completed may be different from those required during the course, the manner of weighing required skills against personal difficulties relies on similar principles.

POINTS TO CONSIDER REGARDING TASKS IN EMPLOYMENT

Few jobs, except perhaps particular pieces of work in a manufacturing industry, consist of only a single task. Most jobs consist of a variety of duties, not all of which are directly connected with the post in which the person is employed. It may be such tasks the person with perceptuo-motor difficulties finds most difficult.

Case note

When Jane took up her first post as a nursery nurse she found that, in addition to dealing with the children in the nursery, she was also expected to prepare their mid-morning drinks. She had always found pouring liquids from any container difficult. The concentrated orange juice which the children drank when diluted was held in plastic, one-gallon containers. Thus it was necessary to pour a small amount of the concentrate into each beaker before water was added.

Jane found this an impossible task and more concentrate was on the work surface than in the beakers! Her therapist suggested to her that she should undertake this task on the draining board of the sink so that any spills could be easily washed away. A second suggestion was that she should first decant the concentrate into a wide topped jug with an accurate pouring lip and pour it into the children's beakers from the jug. These two strategies proved to be helpful not only in helping her to pour more accurately but also in reducing her level of anxiety: she was more confident and her hands were less unsteady.

A person employed to undertake junior clerical duties may also be expected to prepare drinks for other members of staff and carry full cups or beakers to them. This task may prove to be more difficult and cause more anxiety than the one for which the person is actually employed; a sales assistant may be an excellent sales person but have difficulty with the recording necessary for stock control and the like; a therapist may have excellent remedial skills but find ordering data to be stored by microcomputer irritatingly difficult.

It is particularly important for people with perceptuo-motor difficulties to understand exactly what a job entails before the appointment is accepted. A detailed job description is vital.

1. Does the job entail working with other people?
2. Does the job entail organizing other members of staff?
3. Will there be contact with members of the public?
4. Does the work depend on speed or a high degree of accuracy?
5. Is the work repetitive or does each task need to be individually planned?
6. Does the work involve the use of machinery or other mechanical or electrical equipment?
7. Does the work include answering the telephone and recording written messages which must be read by other people?

DRIVING

Many people need to drive to reach their place of employment; some choose to do so rather than travel by public transport. Travel to work takes place for most people during peak hours when most vehicles are on the road. Are there any reasons why people who suffer from perceptuo-motor difficulties should not drive a motor vehicle, especially on congested roads?

People who have obvious physical disabilities will seek advice regarding the advisability of driving a motor vehicle. There are various centres, such as Banstead Place Mobility Centre, which will assess driving ability and advise on vehicle adaptation. Facilities are available where the perceptual skills and reaction times necessary to drive safely on public roads will be assessed. People who have no overt physical disabilities, who suffer only from perceptuo-motor difficulties are unlikely to be advised to attend for assessment at such a centre.

The Highway Code, prepared by the Department of the Environment and the Central Office of Information, mentions the required standard of visual acuity and not driving while under the influence of drugs or alcohol. No mention is made of the need for accurate estimation of speed and distance, reaction times and using more than one control at the same time.

Should people with perceptuo-motor difficulties seek advice before driving on public roads? A headteacher of a school for boys with specific learning difficulties, which often include difficulties with visual perception and gross and fine motor skills, strongly advises his pupils not to ride motor cycles of any description. He does so after many years of experience with such boys and having known a number of them, more than in the general population, to have had one or more accidents, some of them serious. Though his data are not the result of rigorous research, statistically analysed, in the light of his experience, his advice would seem to be wise.

Why do some people seem more prone to road traffic accidents than others? Could it be that those who suffer from perceptuo-motor difficulties are likely to have more accidents than others? Affected people will be able to learn the necessary procedures of driving a motor vehicle and learn the laws of the road. Further skills are required, however, to drive in heavy traffic when it is necessary to have swift reactions to the actions of other drivers and to be able to judge speed and distance. (These are the skills which were discussed previously in relation to difficulties with contact sports). There may be further difficulty with these judgements when driving in the dark.

It is suggested, therefore, that consideration should be given to the assessment of perceptual, kinesthetic and motor planning skills before a full driving licence may be obtained.

7

Strategies within the home and family

> Here's a house
> Here's a door
> Windows, one, two
> Three, four.
>
> *Play School,* BBC Television

Most people, at some time in their lives, live with other people. That group of people may consist of parents and siblings, or a parent living with a partner, with or without children of that partnership or a previous partnership. People also live together because they have chosen to set up a household together or because they have leased a room in a shared house. Some people, either through choice or circumstance, may live alone at some point in their lives.

Whatever the life circumstances, people need a base from which to function. An enclosed area where they may attend to personal hygiene, sleep, prepare and eat food, store personal possessions and be protected from the elements. The sophistication of this personal space will depend on the personal choice of the occupants, financial status, the lifestyle of other people living in the area and that of their peer group. The organization of that living space will also be influenced by the motor and perceptual skills of the occupants.

It is all too easy to appreciate perceptuo-motor difficulties in a clinical setting where assessment or treatment is being carried out. It is more difficult to appreciate that these difficulties are ever-present for the person concerned. That extra bit of conscious effort and attention to tasks, which is relatively simple to apply to activities in a clinical setting is required for every task people with perceptuo-motor difficulties undertake. Maintaining living space and cooperating with others who share that space takes constant effort which is difficult for people without such difficulties to comprehend.

Strategies which will ease the effort required for the skills of daily living and leisure activities will, therefore, be of great help.

ORGANIZATION

Many people with perceptuo-motor difficulties have spent their childhood and adolescent days with their bedroom in chaos. Their ears have rung with exhortations from exasperated parents to put their clothes, toys, magazines, tapes and compact discs away. Lack of organization is often common to all other problems. Probably the majority of parents complain at some time of their children's untidiness. For most children this irritating behaviour disappears with maturity. For the person with perceptuo-motor difficulties it can be a lifelong problem, irritating others and causing frustration in self when a required object is not to hand.

'A place for every thing, and everything in its place' (Simpson, 1985) is a glib saying, but none-the-less one that should not be ignored by those who find organization of living space and possessions difficult. The habit of never putting anything down but always putting it away may seem irksome for the moment, but experience will prove it to be a saver of time and patience in the long run.

Case note

Organization of personal belongings had never been easy for William. As a child his gross motor skills were such that he avoided contact sports. At a fine motor level construction activities which required a high degree of three-dimensional perception were his forte. Those which required precise motor planning such as handwriting were difficult, particularly as they involved prolonged and consistent effort.

As a teenager his room was often ankle deep with discarded garments which had either been worn or taken from his wardrobe and rejected in favour of another garment. Amongst these clothes would be cassette tapes, magazines, tools, receipts, etc. On many occasions a desired object could not be found, so another one was purchased.

William chose a career as an upholsterer. He excels at his job and he is in great demand. The problem with organization persists and in running a business it is a real problem. For the present, the difficulty has been resolved by his relationship with a woman who is happy to organize his home and the paperwork his business involves.

CARE OF THE HOME

People vary in the standard of care they wish to maintain in their home. For some it takes priority over all other activities, for others it is a necessary though not relished part of life. There are, however, basic levels of cleanliness which for comfort and hygiene must be maintained. There are strategies which can be used to ease the extra effort required by those with perceptuo-motor difficulties.

Vacuum cleaners

Machines are broadly of two types, upright and cylinder models. Upright models pick up more dust than cylinder models because they rely on revolving brushes and beater bars in addition to suction. They also give carpets a more 'groomed' appearance. Cylinder models are easier to manoeuvre when cleaning under furniture and on a staircase. Where possible, it is best for the person with perceptuo-motor difficulties to test a number of different machines and make a purchase which causes least problems for them regarding the particular types of difficulty they experience. Decisions about which type of machine will best suit the user can be helped by consulting the results of a 'product test' in *Which?* (Consumer Association Ltd, 1990).

Keeping the cleaner in good working order will ensure that efforts are not wasted. In more recent models of vacuum cleaners, a light is illuminated or a noise is emitted when the dust bag is full. The suction of the machine will be most effective when the dust bag is not over-full. Ensuring that any hose or parts which carry the dust into the bag are not blocked or partially blocked will also ensure efficient functioning.

Organization of a task, sequencing and working methodically are difficulties frequently encountered by people with perceptuo-motor difficulties. These problems can make chores such as vacuum cleaning ineffective and disappointing. Help with the actual method of using a vacuum cleaner effectively are useful. Suggestions such as clearing furniture and working methodically on each area of a floor in turn seem too obvious to be made. However, learning to work methodically can make a world of difference to the time and effort expended and to the satisfaction with the results.

Cleaning surfaces

The suggestions about organization and sequencing discussed when using a vacuum cleaner also apply to cleaning surfaces, whether they are to be polished or washed. Dust clings more readily to a cloth with a fluffy but stable surface than to a completely smooth one. There are cloths made of non-woven synthetic fibres which are ultra-absorbent and useful for mopping up spills of liquids. Cloths which are used wet need to be constructed from absorbant fibres. Again, obvious statements, but for the person who finds household cleaning difficult, suggestions which could improve the results of their efforts.

Clearing a surface before attempting to clean it is a better method than moving objects one at a time and cleaning the part of the surface from which it was moved; the latter method often being adopted by people who have organizational difficulties. Similarly, making a habit of working systematically over a surface will prevent having to return to clean parts which have been missed.

Laundry

Most people today wash their clothes and household linen in a machine, a much simpler task than laundering by hand. The main pitfalls of using a washing machine are sorting clothes into groups which can be safely washed together, and judging the correct weight of items with which to load the machine. An over-heavy load will put strain on the machine and a load which is too tightly packed will prevent the items from rotating and so they will not be adequately cleaned. Some items, particularly clothing, need to be hand-washed.

The following points will help people who have difficulty judging weight, volume and washability, to launder items satisfactorily.

1. Have to hand a list of the symbols used to indicate laundering procedures so that it may be easily referred to when reading garment labels. Care should be taken to ensure that the correct washing and spin drying cycle is chosen for different fabrics. Synthetic fabrics will be unnecessarily creased if they are spun for too long or at too high a speed.

2. Look at garment labels before a purchase is made to ensure that the item is machine washable. It is expensive to have clothes dry cleaned; this may often be required for people who are apt to let drips from cups, fragments of food or splashes of other substances mark their clothes.

3. If there is difficulty judging a suitable volume of load, using a suitable sized basket into which items may be 'measured' before putting them in the machine may be helpful.

4. If necessary, weigh the basket of clothes on bathroom scales to ensure that the load is not too heavy. After checking the weight a number of times, it will become easier to judge without weighing. Instructions supplied with washing machines often include a list of the approximate weights of items such as sheets and towels and may also suggest selections of items which will make a suitable load.

5. Bright or dark colours should be separated from white or very light coloured items. Regarding coloured items, if in doubt do not put it in the load!

6. Different fabrics, of course, require washing at different temperatures. In addition, some synthetics become permanently creased if spun dry at too high a speed. Erring on the side of caution is best. Choose the correct temperature and spin speed for the most delicate item in the load. Items which are still very wet when taken

from the machine can be spun dry again but permanent creases cannot be easily removed.

7. Because it is often necessary to launder clothes frequently, fabrics which require the minimum of ironing are most suitable. Cotton and synthetic mixtures are easier to iron than 100% cotton ones. Tucks, frills and pleats complicate ironing.

8. Items ironed as soon as they are line dry will require less work on them than those which have been dried and left folded for some time.

9. Tumble dryers are useful when clothes cannot be dried outside but they are an expensive way of completely drying laundry. A tumble dryer which signals the end of a pre-set drying period will prevent clothes being over-dried. Fabrics which have become snuff dry will be difficult to iron.

10. Tumble dryers are also very useful for people who find ironing difficult to accomplish satisfactorily. If clothes from the washing machine are tumbled in a dryer for 5 minutes before hanging to dry completely many of the creases will be removed and most fabrics will take far less effort to iron.

Many of these points seem all too obvious but for the person with difficulty making such judgements they may need to be carefully considered a number of times until the required judgements are learned.

Step ladders

For people who do not have a clear perception of their position in space, unless they are giving it conscious consideration, step ladders can be a hazard. Everyone should take care when using them; the following points are particularly important for people with spatial difficulties.

1. Always use a step ladder when appropriate; do not try to balance precariously on unstable stools, chairs or tables.

2. Ensure that the step ladder is in good condition, that it does not wobble as it is mounted and that all its joints are secure.

3. Use a step ladder which has treads sufficiently large to support a good proportion of the feet.

4. Choose a step ladder which has a platform at the top with plenty of room for standing and slight adjustment of the position of the feet.
5. A step ladder with a rail above the top platform makes a helpful hand grip and prevents the user accidentally walking off the platform.
6. A step stool is useful for reaching up to high shelves. A kickstool fitted with spring-loaded castors, immobilized when weight is on the stool, forms a large, stable base on which to stand. The two treads are covered with non-slip rubberized material (Figure 7.1)

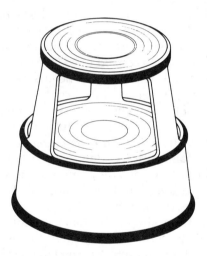

Figure 7.1 A kickstool which is an easily moveable yet stable means of reaching items stored on high shelves, etc.

Cooking

Any cooking process is potentially dangerous. It involves dealing with sources of intense heat, hot liquids, fats and foods. Kitchens are often the most congested area of a home with members of the household gravitating to this focal point. Therefore there may be many sources of distraction for the person who is cooking. There are basic rules which apply to everyone who uses a kitchen and special precautions which should be taken by those who have difficulty with motor planning, motor control and spatial difficulties.

1. Equipment in the kitchen should be arranged so that there is no need to reach across pans or other receptacles containing hot liquid.
2. There should be a suitable surface adjacent to the cooker where hot items may be safely placed.
3. The handles of pans should be turned away from the edge of the cooker so that they cannot be accidentally caught by a hand or clothing and the hot contents of the pan spilled.
4. A colander should be used when draining vegetables which have been boiled in water. There is danger of scalding the arm with rising steam if the lid of the saucepan is used as a draining device. A safer system is to use a mesh basket to hold the vegetables inside the pan. This enables the vegetables when cooked to be lifted from the saucepan in the basket, thus removing the need to carry the saucepan to remove the water until it is cool.
5. Most items of food can be moved in a hot frying pan more easily with tongs than with a spatula or fish slice. Sausages are easier to turn if, before cooking, they are pinned together in pairs with wooden (not plastic) cocktail sticks. Because they are in pairs they have flat surfaces rather than rounded ones and therefore do not roll about in the pan.
6. A food processor can remove the need to chop foods such as onions. Care should be taken to follow the manufacturer's instructions. In particular, the machine must be turned off before attempting to remove the lid. The pusher, never the hand, must always be used to ease food down the tube. Washing the processor will require a brush to ensure that all particles of food have been removed. It is better not to put the sharp blades in water with other items to be washed, to prevent cuts. For the same reason, a brush with a handle is the best tool for cleaning the blades.
7. Kitchen knives should be stored separately from other kitchen tools so that they are less likely to cause accidental injury.
8. Kitchen scissors, though not approved of by many chefs, are often a safer means of cutting some foods such as chicken joints than a knife.

As with many other activities people with perceptuo-motor difficulties will cope better in the kitchen if they make a conscious effort to organize equipment and their own activity systematically. Often, total concentration is required and working slowly usually leads to a task being accomplished with the least problems and often more quickly and satisfactorily.

SEWING AND OTHER HANDIWORK

Many people who suffer from various combinations of perceptuo-motor difficulties would like to undertake some type of needlecraft or already do so but experience a number of difficulties.

Scissors

It is important for left-handed people to have scissors which are constructed to be used in a left-handed manner. This enables the left-handed user to have a better view of the line along which the cut will be made and that the blades are being forced together, and not apart, when cutting. On large dressmaking shears this also ensures that the angle of the handles into which the thumb is inserted moulds round the base of the thumb and that its edge is not causing pressure on the metacarpo-phalangeal joint.

For people who cannot readily undertake rhythmical apposition of the thumb to fingers sprung, whole-hand-grip scissors will be easier to manipulate. These scissors require whole-hand flexion to operate them; the scissors are opened by releasing the grip on them and allowing their spring device to come into action. There are also very small snipping scissors available which fit into the palm of the hand with a ring to accommodate one finger. These scissors require an even smaller palmar movement (Figure 7.2 and Appendix B).

It is important to have the correct type of scissors for the task to be undertaken. Intricate cutting with many changes of direction requires small, usually pointed scissors, whereas cutting long, straight lines requires long-bladed scissors to facilitate long, smooth cuts. The weight and strength of scissors should also be related to the weight of the material being cut.

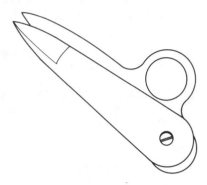

Figure 7.2 Palmar grip scissors which require only a small whole hand movement. They are sprung to open automatically when the grip is released.

Some people benefit not only from the above suggestions, but also from having guidance with cutting techniques. Pointing out that the technique for cutting intricate curved shapes requires as much effort and movement of the hand which is holding the material, as of the cutting hand. The scissors should make very small cuts synchronized with the small adjustments of the position of the material in the other hand.

When cutting out a garment previous to sewing it there is usually a paper pattern pinned to the material. This type of cutting requires long cuts to be made along the length of the blade of the scissors. The person cutting should arrange themselves so that the non-cutting hand steadies the pattern on the paper and ensure that it does not move whilst cutting.

Arranging paper patterns on material

Perceptual difficulties, particularly those related to position in space and spatial relationships can cause problems when laying out pattern pieces on material. Consideration of several points will help to circumvent such difficulties.

1. Study the selection of pattern layouts on the instruction leaflet supplied with the pattern. Circle clearly with a pen the appropriate layout according to the size of the garment being made and the width of the material.
2. Select the pattern pieces required for the version of the garment being made. Put any pieces not required away in the pattern envelope. Iron the paper pattern pieces to remove creases so that their shape is not distorted.
3. Lay out the material on a large table or on the floor, folding the material as indicated on the pattern layout. Ensure that any fold of the material and selvedges are in the same orientation as on the layout plan. This last suggestion is very important for people who have difficulty with spatial orientation.
4. Lay out the pattern pieces on the material as suggested on the layout plan, at least until the experience has been gained in cutting out patterns.
5. The pieces can be pinned more accurately if the points of the pins are inserted so that they point towards the edges of the pattern pieces.

Sewing machines

Once the technique of using a sewing machine has been mastered it will probably produce better results than hand sewing. The latter requires even, rhythmical movements of the needle as well as accurate judgement of exactly where the needle should be inserted in the fabric. A sewing machine removes the need for these skills though, of course, different skills are needed in order to be able to use a sewing machine effectively.

1. It is important to become familiar with the model of machine being used, including how to oil it, keep it dust and lint free and adjust the tension. New sewing machines are supplied with a detailed instruction book and some suppliers offer free lessons following purchase.
2. Ensure that the correct needle is used for the fabric being sewn. Some fabrics, such as tricot, are best sewn with a ballpoint needle. Discard needles which are bent or blunt and those which have developed a burr on the tip.

3. Use a thread to suit the fabric being sewn. Usually natural fibres are best sewn with a cotton thread and synthetics with synthetic thread. There are exceptions to this rule, for example very fine silk fabric is often better sewn with a fine synthetic thread; natural silk thread may be too heavy.
4. Adjust the stitch length according to the fabric being sewn. Generally, the heavier the fabric the longer the stitch length which is suitable.
5. Tacking/basting before machine sewing will save the heartache of unpicking a resultant poorly fitting garment.
6. Iron or press each seam immediately after it has been sewn or at least before it is crossed by the sewing of another seam. A good rule is to set up the iron and ironing board every time the sewing machine is to be used.
7. Until experience has been gained, follow the sewing guide which is provided with all paper patterns.

PHOTOGRAPHS

Perceptual difficulties can cause problems both with taking photographs and having photographs taken. Photographs of some people never seem to depict how they appear in real life. Photographs taken by some people often have the people or objects badly placed in the photographic frame or parts have been unintentionally cut off the top, bottom or sides of the photograph.

People who are left-handed may have a further problem, for camera parts are arranged to suit right-handed people. It may be possible to use some cameras upside-down so that parts are more conveniently placed to be used by a left-handed person.

Taking photographs

1. Familiarity with the camera being used will help those with spatial difficulties.
2. Position the subject within the viewfinder so that they are seen to be comfortably within the edges of the frame. This is because the resultant photograph will usually be a little smaller than that seen through the viewfinder. Most

cameras show a frame a little within the edges of the viewfinder, within which the subject of the photograph should be placed.

3. Some people are able to focus the camera effectively but spoil their efforts when actually taking the photograph by moving the camera as they concentrate on depressing the shutter release button or even simply by breathing. A suggestion from a press photographer which may be helpful is to breathe in and hold the breath whilst actually taking the photograph.

4. People with perceptuo-motor difficulties usually obtain better results if they take photographs of static subjects. Taking a photograph of a moving object requires the photographer to focus the camera and press the shutter release button almost simultaneously. This can cause similar types of difficulties to playing contact games where problems are encountered in attempting to employ a number of strategies simultaneously.

5. An instamatic camera, which requires the photographer only to 'aim and shoot', is the simplest type to use. It eliminates the need for adjustments to the lens, shutter speed, etc., leaving the photographer free to give complete attention to framing the picture.

Having a photograph taken

People who have problems with appreciation of body image and position in space often find that posed photographs of themselves are disappointing. Snapshots where the person being photographed is unaware that a photograph is being taken are often more pleasing.

One solution to the problem is to use a very skilled photographer who will allow plenty of time for a session and has some skill not only with a camera but also with handling people. Having a friend or relative at the session who is able to distract the subject from the camera and encourage relaxation may be helpful as is a little humour introduced into the occasion.

Preparing for the photographic session by arranging the hair in a flattering style and applying a make-up which flatters the features and minimizes faults, where applicable, will not only improve the resultant photographs but also increase the confidence of the sitter. Clothes which enhance the figure are also helpful. For instance, choose a shirt or blouse which is becoming to the face and neck. The shoulder line is defined and neatened by small shoulder pads if suitable for the garment being worn.

A tip from a professional photographer to help relax the muscles of the face is to close the eyes for a short while and have the photographer take the photograph when he/she tells the subject to open the eyes.

PHYSICAL LEISURE ACTIVITIES

Most people gravitate towards leisure activities which give them pleasure, in the short or long term, and to those at which they can participate with a fair degree of competency.

Arriving at such choices for people with perceptuo-motor difficulties may not be a smooth path. For example, a person may take an instinctive delight in dance but suffer from spatial and rhythmic difficulties which prevent active participation. Similar difficulties may preclude musical activities. A career on the stage or an interest in amateur dramatics may be frustrated by a poor sense of body image, spatial difficulties or poor memory which makes learning a script accurately a problem. (There are, of course, those who have enjoyed a successful career on the stage despite the last difficulty.) Such an interest may be satisfied with behind-the-scenes activity in the theatre.

In these circumstances it is all too easy for people to become spectators rather than participators. Sport on television, taped music or that broadcast on the radio may become fanatical interests to the exclusion of active leisure pursuits. Careful assessment of strengths and weaknesses can enable most people to discover active leisure pursuits with which they may meet with an acceptable degree of satisfaction.

1. Slowness of response to the actions of others may preclude contact sports such as soccer, hockey or netball. For example a person may be perfectly capable of catching a ball which is being thrown and caught reciprocally between self and another person. However if a game requires

instant readiness to catch a ball thrown from an unpre-determined angle over an unplanned distance it may not be possible to respond by adjusting position and preparing to catch in the time available.

2. There are a number of sporting activities in which time is not of the essence, such as golf, archery, darts, swimming and field sports. In such sports the participant has no need to react swiftly to the action of others. It is an acceptable element of such activities that time is taken to arrange the bodily position and pre-plan movements including power, speed and direction. People with perceptuo-motor problems will be more likely to enjoy such activities and meet with an acceptable degree of success than in contact sports.

3. Many people take part in activities which are designed to promote physical fitness. Such exercise can take a number of forms and it would be inappropriate here to discuss the advantages and disadvantages of the various types of activity. People with perceptuo-motor difficulties will, however, meet with greater success in activities which do not rely on speed, complex sequences of movement or sustaining a pre-set rhythm particularly in unison with a group of other people.

Many people who suffer from perceptuo-motor difficulties have found participation in the sporting activities available within school difficult. Organization of staff time and sports' facilities often make activities other than team games imprac-tical. Such people may have developed a distaste for all physical activities and become reluctant to participate in more suitable activities in adult life. Because of the likelihood of the development of poor posture and limited use of muscle groups it is important for such people to find some form of physical activity with which they feel comfortable and able to sustain a continuing interest.

Case note

Sarah had been referred to a child development centre at 4 years of age. Assessment showed that she was of average intellectual level but had severe perceptuo-motor difficulties.

These difficulties affected her integration of sensory input, gross and fine motor ability and her ability to comprehend and express language.

She continued to attend the centre with her mother. A physiotherapist, speech therapist and occupational therapist proceeded with a programme of treatment in which her parents were very much involved. Her therapists discussed her special needs with her school teachers who took into account her difficulties when planning her educational programme.

At 11 years of age it was decided that Sarah would benefit from spending an extra year at primary school. Thus, at 17 years of age she is just now beginning to prepare for her GCSE examinations.

Considering her original and residual difficulties, with the help of her admirable parents she has made remarkable progress. With remedial help she has remained in mainstream school. She has spent several holidays away from home without her parents with supervised peer groups. She is able to travel into her home town centre and make appropriate purchases from shops. Most commendable, as a guide she was successful in gaining the Baden Powell award, the highest award made in the movement.

Sarah is a very tall girl, 5 feet 11 inches, and on a recent visit to see her therapist her mother mentioned her tendency to stoop. This, of course commonly occurs in tall adolescents. Attempts to remediate this stoop revealed that one of her original problems, dyspraxia, was still evident. She was unable to voluntarily and consciously retract her shoulders. Suggestions have been made as to how Sarah can improve her posture, though her residual difficulties are making this a difficult task.

This anecdote illustrates the far-reaching effects of perceptuo-motor difficulties and the importance of suitable forms of physical exercise for such people.

PERSONAL AND SEXUAL RELATIONSHIPS

Much has been written and discussed about the personal and sexual relationships of people with physical disability or learning difficulties (mental handicap). One of the main means by which this has taken place in Britain is SPOD, the Association to Aid the Sexual and Personal Relationships of People with a Disability. The organization produces a number of leaflets, resource lists and books. It also arranges courses, some organized to suit the participant's particular needs.

Information and help is not so readily available for people who suffer from perceptuo-motor difficulties. There is no doubt that their needs are not so great as for those who, because of severe physical disability, find social contact difficult and sexual relationships restricted. Nevertheless perceptuo-motor difficulties must affect social and sexual relationships.

Research has shown that not all perceptuo-motor difficulties of childhood resolve with maturity (Shelley and Reister, 1972; Gillberg and Gillberg, 1989; Losse *et al.*, 1991). There are adults who continue to suffer from this type of difficulty, some of which will have been diagnosed and perhaps also treated during childhood years. There is an even larger number of adults whose problems have never been formally diagnosed.

Considering the effects which perceptuo-motor difficulties can have on almost any facet of life, it is not unreasonable to infer that they will have an effect on developing and sustaining social relationships.

Posture and the way clothes are worn contribute to the initial impression given to others and attractiveness in the eyes of others. Similarly, the manner in which a person walks and moves gives an often unconscious impression to other people. Tempering of the voice, grading of a smile, a laugh or other reaction impresses others. The choice of paid work and leisure activities will affect the number of people who are encountered and their personalities.

There are also the effects of perceptuo-motor difficulties on self to consider. People may have a poor self-image, perhaps because of lack of gracefulness, poor sporting ability or self-consciousness on a dance floor. This may result in reserve in situations where people meet together. This poor self-image and lack of self-confidence may also influence sense of value as a person, having an effect on the choice, conscious or unconscious of friends and social associates.

Much more tenuous is the suggestion that perceptuo-motor difficulties have adverse effects on sexual relationships.

Because sexual relationships are unlikely to be precluded by even the severest types of perceptuo-motor difficulties it is unlikely that professional help will be sought directly as a result of them. It may be, however, that some problems associated with sexual relationships may have, at their root, difficulties of a perceptuo-motor nature. Dissatisfaction between partners may arise because one or both partners have difficulty with position in space of self or partner and spatial relationships between the two. Difficulties may also arise because of poor sense of rhythm or ability to anticipate the reaction or movements of a partner.

Would it be helpful in such situations if everyone with perceptuo-motor difficulties were aware of the nature of their difficulties? Would it be of additional help if partners were equally aware of them? Therapists and others who counsel people on problems with sexual relationships certainly should be aware of the possibility of perceptuo-motor difficulties being a significant element of their problems.

CHILDBIRTH

The experience of childbirth is a very personal event for each woman concerned. Medical attitudes to the event change with the passage of years as do the philosophies of midwives, doctors and obstetricians. Much attention is now given to the preparation of the expectant mother, and often the father too, for childbirth. Courses are designed to prepare the woman's body for the event, explain the process of childbirth and encourage the woman's participation in the process.

Could it be that women who suffer from perceptuo-motor difficulties should be given particular attention and extra help both before and during childbirth? It may be that problems with coordination, sequencing and rhythm could have an effect on both the first and second stages of labour. These difficulties may be particularly significant during the active second stage of labour when muscle contraction must be coordinated with the force necessary to expel the child.

These suggestions are tentative, though it seems reasonable that women who have perceptuo-motor problems which cause difficulties in other areas of life could also find that they affect childbirth. Extra help during the prenatal period together with special consideration from obstetric staff during childbirth could make this time more satisfying for such women.

CHILD-CARE

No amount of guidance and instruction can prepare prospective parents adequately for parenthood. Prior to the event it is difficult to imagine that such a small person can take over the life of at least one person. Theory of how to bath a baby or change a nappy is very different in practice when that baby is ones own precious wriggling bundle. People with perceptuo-motor difficulties may be particularly apprehensive, particularly in the days of caring for a new baby. There are a few basic points which may help parents in such a situation.

1. While the baby is in a safe place such as a cot or pram, make all the necessary preparations for bathing, changing or feeding the baby.
2. It is helpful to keep all the necessary equipment together. For example, items required for changing a nappy are best kept together in a container which can easily be moved to whichever part of the house it may be needed.
3. It is very important to have all the required equipment very near to hand when bathing the baby; one hand will be needed to hold the baby, so that only one hand will be free to deal with equipment.
4. A wet baby can be very slippery. A small towel or terry nappy in the bottom of the bath will provide a degree of friction to help prevent slipping. Holding the baby by placing one arm behind its head and firmly grasping the baby's upper arm with that hand will ensure that the baby is held securely.
5. Should a parent be nervous about walking downstairs whilst holding the baby, the use of a baby sling at such times will be helpful and reassuring. It is inadvisable to carry anything else other than the baby when walking downstairs.

Most people with perceptuo-motor difficulties will, given time, discover their own strategies for coping with a young baby. As children become more independent, coping with their physical needs will be simpler. Other areas of the parent/child relationship may become more difficult when the concommitants of perceptuo-motor difficulties are considered.

Difficulties with organization, consistency, self-confidence and self-esteem which often accompany perceptuo-motor difficulties could affect some parent's ability to handle their children. Such people may need to make conscious efforts to provide their children with consistency of handling and help with organizing play, personal space and life-skills.

8

Conclusions

It is not enough to understand what we ought to be,
unless we know what we are; and we do not understand
what we are, unless we know what we ought to be.
                                        T.S. Eliot, 1935

Perceptuo-motor difficulties do not create world headlines,
though of late the press has given more lineage to the problem
if only in the form of feature articles and brief reports on current
research. The population in general does not view such
difficulties as a cause for great concern. They are not life-
threatening, nor can they be cured by heroic surgery.

Perhaps there is most interest in perceptuo-motor difficulties
when symptoms occur together with reading, writing and/or
spelling difficulties when the combination of symptoms may
be labelled dyslexia. Lexical problems, difficulty in attaining
acceptable standards of reading, handwriting and spelling, are
usually considered more significant in today's literate world.
It is not widely appreciated what far-reaching effects perceptuo-
motor difficulties can have on the life of the sufferer, even in
the absence of any specific difficulty with encoding and
decoding the written word. By and large, parents of a child
who is coping with academic subjects in school but has poor
gross motor skills will show less concern than parents of a child
who is agile but is having difficulty learning to read.

Since the 1960s, however, there has been increasing interest
on the part of therapists and paediatricians in the diagnosis
and treatment of perceptuo-motor difficulties. Physiotherapists, occupational therapists, orthoptists and speech and
language therapists have shared their specialist skills to the

benefit of such children. This medical and paramedical interest has stimulated the interest of educationalists into the difficulties such children experience.

Gradually children who are reluctant to take part in physical education and games lessons are being investigated, lest they prove to have specific difficulty with gross motor skills. It is now realized that children who produce only small amounts of handwriting may not be lazy or lacking in application but may have fine motor or motor planning difficulties. In a similar way, children who begin a piece of work with even and legible handwriting, but deteriorate into an illegible scrawl at the bottom of the page, may be expending their maximum effort and resolve. Today the difficulties under which these children complete only a small amount of handwriting is more likely to be appreciated. The words 'must make more effort with written work' are appearing less frequently on end-of-term reports.

Considering the small numbers of children who are examined by paediatricians and who take part in treatment programmes devised by therapists, only a small percentage of children with perceptuo-motor difficulties are receiving the attention from which they could benefit. Research has suggested that between 5 and 10% of children suffer from some degree of such difficulties (Henderson and Hall, 1982; Roussounis, Gaussen and Stratton, 1987). A large number of children must remain undiagnosed and perhaps some are living under the shadow of being suspected of having only limited ability. A major means of communication from pupil to teacher remains by pen and paper and thus the child who has undiagnosed difficulty with handwriting may be underestimated on a daily basis.

Understandably some children who suffer from perceptuo-motor difficulties also have behavioural problems. Researchers who have taken a second look, after an interval of a number of years, have found that a proportion of their subjects have developed emotional and behavioural problems (Gillberg and Gillberg, 1989; Losse *et al.*, 1991). Personal observation of younger children has noted such problems occurring together with perceptuo-motor difficulties. Whether these behavioural problems result from the unsympathetic treatment of perceptuo-motor difficulties, occur in the same child as independent problems or if the behavioural difficulties are a further manifestation of perceptuo-motor problems, is not proven. It could be that causes of behavioural problems are specific to each individual child with the possibilty that there are multiple causes.

Again, personal experience has suggested that children manifest fewer behavioural problems if their strengths and weaknesses are assessed, the conclusions are explained to the child's parents and teachers, and realistic strategies are devised to help them learn the skills necessary for daily life. Perhaps even more important is to explain to the child in appropriate language the reasons why some skills are difficult to accomplish. A discussion with the child of which activities are important to her/him is also helpful. It must be stressed to both the child and parents that the child is loved and valued as a person no matter what difficulties are encountered. These strategies often help to diffuse a potentially explosive situation.

To date most interest has been shown in the perceptuo-motor difficulties of childhood. Interest was first focused on junior school children who experienced difficulty in the classroom. Of late, increasing interest is being shown in diagnosing the possibility of problems in younger children so that, when possible, they may be averted and when necessary any special educational needs may be anticipated. The large proportion of references cited in this book which refer to research undertaken with infant and junior school children illustrates the concentration of interest in this age group.

Some early researchers stressed the benefit of intervention (Dare and Gordon, 1970). They could only know in retrospect how long remedial programmes needed to be sustained and if improvement was maintained after cessation of remediation. Personal experience suggests that these children need continuing support throughout the changing manifestations of perceptuo-motor problems throughout school days.

Researchers are now beginning to look again at adolescents who, as children, were diagnosed as having perceptuo-motor difficulties. Some conclude that only those children with severe problems continue to be affected by them in adolescence (Knuckey and Gubbey, 1983). A more recent study suggests that it is erroneous to believe that such children will 'grow out of' their difficulties. A large proportion of adolescents in this study continued to experience motor difficulties, in addition to problems with social and emotional adaptation (Losse *et al.*, 1991). The latter appeared to have a greater effect on their lives than actual perceptuo-motor difficulties.

Does promotion to adulthood mysteriously lead to the resolution of perceptuo-motor difficulties and their concomitants? The paucity of medical and paramedical literature would lead one to believe that this is so. Listening to the comments of lay people would suggest the opposite. Comments of the following types often point to unacknowledged perceptuo-motor difficulties in adults.

- 'He/she is no good with his/her hands.'
- 'It takes me an hour to decipher a letter from him/her.'
- 'He/she does not anticipate having to stop at traffic lights when driving a car.'
- 'Their windows never look clean, there are always parts they have not wiped.'
- 'You should see the mess when he/she is cooking, spills everywhere and every pot and pan in the house is dirty.'
- 'Her make-up never looks right, she always has more eyeshadow on one eye than the other and her lipstick is never even.'

For most adults with perceptuo-motor difficulties the pattern of life is established. Family, friends and colleagues are likely to have accepted behaviour in the affected individual as their 'norm'. The individual themselves may have become resigned to their own difficulties though not necessarily be content to live with them. Frustration may be felt because of desired goals which are impossible to attain.

Only medical and paramedical practitioners who are conversant with perceptuo-motor difficulties are likely to recognize them as such in adults. Adults with perceptuo-motor difficulties, even if they are recognized are unlikely to be referred for investigation and treatment. Perhaps it should be regarded as a bonus if these difficulties are appreciated and handled sympathetically when they are recognized in people who are consulting medical and paramedical practitioners about other medical or surgical problems.

The following are medical situations which may arouse suspicion of perceptuo-motor difficulties:

1. The patient who is unable to coordinate swallowing in order to take a tablet or capsule.
2. The patient who is unable to coordinate activating a spinhaler with breathing in order to take the required dose.
3. The patient who has difficulty learning to use crutches probably because of poor sequential skills and difficulty with maintaining the rhythm of the movement of crutches and leg.
4. The dental patient who experiences a gag reflex when the dentist is working at the back of the mouth or is taking an impression with an alginate compound prior to making a denture.
5. The patient who is difficult to position for X-rays.
6. The patient who has difficulty 'moving with' the physiotherapist during a treatment session.

During recent years there has been research undertaken studying the relationship between the existence of soft neurological signs and psychiatric illness. In a study of adolescents who had a diagnosis of anxiety-withdrawal symptoms, 80% of the girls and all the boys earlier had shown neurological soft signs (Shaffer *et al.*, 1985). In an annotation (Shaffer, 1978) various studies are cited which suggest a relationship between neurological dysfunction resulting in delayed milestones, learning problems in school, diagnosed in childhood which were followed by schizophrenic and personality disorders in adult life. Clearly much more research must be undertaken before these links become clearer.

By and large most adults will find their own coping strategies. Some will be philosophical regarding their difficulties and accept them as inevitable. Others will spend a lifetime striving to overcome them. Some will have lifelong regrets that a specific career or leisure pursuit was and continues to be unattainable; the frustrated dancer, actor or sports man or woman. Some will have resolved their frustration in vicarious satisfaction by becoming a loyal spectator of sport or fanatical theatre-goer.

How helpful it would be if knowledge of perceptuo-motor difficulties and their effects on the life of the affected individual was a part of everyone's education. The affected individuals would understand the nature of their own difficulties. They would be much more able to set realistic goals for themselves. Many emotional and behavioural problems could be avoided. The population in general would, over the years, have more understanding of and sympathy towards individuals who suffer from perceptuo-motor difficulties.

Whether or not people with perceptuo-motor difficulties have their problems openly acknowledged or the sufferer is unaware of the nature of their difficulties, they should be assured of several points regarding self. Efforts should be made to ensure that all such people are aware of them regardless of their degree of difficulty, intellectual level or station in life.

'TO WHOM IT MAY CONCERN'

1. No matter how perceptuo-motor problems affect a person, they do not detract in any way from his/her value as a person. Everyone is valuable as a person no matter what their strengths and weaknesses may be.
2. Perceptuo-motor difficulties do not preclude underlying intellectual brightness. Such difficulties affect people with all levels of intellectual ability.
3. Acknowledging problems and appreciating how they can affect all aspects of life is a useful coping strategy.
4. The understanding and constructive assistance of family, friends and colleagues can be very helpful.
5. Accepting self, including any perceptuo-motor difficulties, helps to form a realistic attitude towards self and life events.
6. Accepting and admiring in others skills not possessed by self is a healthy attitude.
7. Though it may be difficult to believe at times, there are many other people who have similar problems.
8. Perceptuo-motor difficulties often mean that the sufferer will have to make a little bit more effort than is necessary for the average person with many everyday activities and most certainly when acquiring new skills. The need to make this extra effort is continuing.

References

Alston, J. and Taylor, J. (1985) *Helping Lefthanded Children with Hand-writing: Interpreting Research for Teachers and Therapists* (Supplement to *The Handwriting File*) LDA, Wisbech, Cambs, UK.

Ayres, A.J. (1972) *Southern California Sensory Integration Test* Western Psychological Services, Los Angeles.

Ayres, A.J. (1974) *The Development of Sensory Integrative Theory and Practice*, p. 161, Kendall/Hunt Publishing Company, Dubuque, I o w a .

Bishop, D. V. M. (1990) *Handedness and Developmental Disorder, Clinics in Developmental Medicine No. 110*, pp. 92 – 100, Mac Keith Press, Blackwell Scientific, London.

Brewer, E.C. (1978) *The Dictionary of Phrase and Fable*, p. 463, Avenel Books, New York.

Briggs, D. (1980) A study of the influence of handwriting upon grades using examination scripts, *Educational Review*, Volume 32, No. 2, 185–93.

Brown, B. and Henderson, S. (1989) A sloping desk? Should the wheel turn full circle? *Handwriting Review*, No. 3, pp 55–9.

Chasty, H. T. (1986) *Handwriting. A Suitable Approach for the Child with Difficulty* Lecture/Handwriting Interest group.

Chesson, R., McKay, C. and Stephenson, E. (1990) Motor/learning difficulties and the family, *Child: Care, Health and Development*, **16**, 123–38.

Clark, M.M. (1970) *Reading Difficulties in Schools*, pp. 45–6, Penguin Books, London.

Consumer Association Ltd (1990) Vacuum cleaners *Which?* May, pp. 276–9.

Corso, J.F. (1970) *The Experimental Psychology of Sensory Behaviour*, pp. 145–55, Holt, Rinehart and Winston, London and New York.

Dare, M.T. and Gordon, N. (1970) Clumsy children: A disorder of perception and motor organisation, *Developmental Medicine and Child Neurology*, **12**, 178–85.

Eliot, T.S. (1935) Religion and Literature in *The International Thesaurus* of Quotations compiled by Tripp, R.T. (1976) p. 577, Penguin Books, London.

Enstrom, E. A. (1962) The extent of the use of the left hand in handwriting, *Journal of Educational Research*, **55**, No. 5, 234–5.

Francis-Williams, J. (1970) *Children with Specific Learning Difficulties*, pp. 57–8, Pergamon Press, Oxford.

Frankenburg, W. K. and Dodds, J. B. (1969) *Denver Developmental Screening Test*, University of Colorado Medical Centre, Denver.

Frostig, M. (1966) *The Marianne Frostig Developmental Test of Visual Perception* Consulting Psychologists Press, Palo Alto, California.

Frostig, M. and Horne, D. (1964) *The Frostig Program for the Development of Visual Perception*, Follet, Chicago.

Gillberg, I. C. and Gillberg, C. (1989) Children with preschool minor neurodevelopmental disorders. IV: Behaviour and school achievement at Age 13, *Developmental Medicine and Child Neurology*, **31**, 3–13.

Gillberg I.C., Gillberg, C. and Groth, J. (1989) Children with preschool minor neurodevelopmental disorders. V: Neurodevelopmental Profiles at Age 13, *Developmental Medicine and Child Neurology*, **31**, 14–24.

Handley, J. (1986a) Posture education in primary schools, *Health at School*, **1**, No 6, 176–7.

Handley, J. (1986b) Posture education in primary schools. Part 2 – Re-education, *Health at School* **1**, No. 7, 220–1.

Handley, J. (1986c) Posture education in primary schools. Part 3 – Reinforcement and assessment, *Health at School*, **1**, No. 8, 259–60.

Hayward, J. F. (1957) *English Cutlery: Sixteenth to Eighteenth Century*, pp. 7–8, Her Majesty's Stationery Office, London.

Henderson, S. E. (1987) The assessment of 'clumsy' children: Old and new approaches, *Journal of Child Psychology and Psychiatry*, **28**, No. 4, 511–27.

Henderson, S. E. and Hall, D. (1982) Concomitants of clumsiness in young schoolchildren, *Developmental Medicine and Child Neurology*, **24**, 448–60.

Hulme, C. and Lord, R. (1986) Clumsy children – a review of recent research, *Child: Care, Health and Development*, **12**, No. 4, 257–69.

Huxley, A. (1931) Music at Night, in *The International Thesaurus of Quotations* compiled by Tripp, R. T. (1970), p. 402, Penguin Books, London.

Illingworth, R. S. (1983) *The Development of the Infant and Young Child: Normal and Abnormal*, 7th edn, p. 152, Churchill Livingstone, Edinburgh and London.

Illingworth, R. S. and Illingworth, C. (1984) *Babies and Young Children A Guide for Parents*, p. 116, Churchill Livingstone, Edinburgh and London.

Jackson, C. (1980) *Colour Me Beautiful*, Acropolis Books, Washington

DC (Judy Piathus (Publishers) Ltd, London, 1983).

Jarman, C. (1984) *Pre-handwriting activities for young children, Gnosis,* No. 5, 26–8.

Jarman, C. (1989) A mythology of handwriting teaching, *Handwriting Review* No. 3, 62–3.

Johnston, O. Short, H. and Crawford, J. (1987) Poorly coordinated children: a survey of 95 cases, *Child: Health, Care and Development,* **13**, 361–76.

Jones, E. G. (1973) *Children Growing up,* p. 121, Penguin Books, London.

Knuckey, N. W. and Gubbay, S. S. (1983) Clumsy children: a prognostic study, *Australian Paediatric Journal,* **19**, 9–13.

Laszlo, J., Bairstow, P. and Bartrip, J. (1988) A new approach to treatment of perceptuo-motor dysfunction: previously called clumsiness. *Support for Learning,* **3**, No. 1, 35–40.

Lewis, C.M. and Salway, A. (1989) Are you sitting comfortably? *Handwriting Review,* 51–4.

Losse, A., Henderson S.E., Elliman, D. *et al.* (1991) Clumsiness in children – do they grow out of it?' *Developmental Medicine and Child Neurology,* **33**, 55–68.

Lyle, J.G. and Johnson, E. G. (1976) Development of lateral consistency and its relation to reading and reversals, *Perceptual and Motor Skills,* **43**, No. 3, Part 1, 695–8.

McKinlay, I. (1987) Children with motor learning difficulties: not so much a syndrome – more a way of life' *Physiotherapy* **73**, No. 11, 635–8.

Maslow, P., Frostig, M., Lefever, W.D. and Whittlesey, J.R. B. (1963) *Developmental Test of Visual Perception. 1963 Standardisation* Consulting Psychologists Press, Palo Alto, California.

Millidot, M. (1986) *Dictionary of Optometry,* p. 121, Butterworth, London.

Moliere (1661) 'The School for Husbands' in *The International Thesaurus of Quotations* compiled by Tripp, R.T. (1976), p. 265, Penguin Books, London.

Oglivie, E. (1978) Training body awareness in the clumsy child, *British Journal of Occupational Therapy,* **41**, No. 7, 233–6.

Page, S. and MacAuslan, A. (1978) Poor handwriting and the pencil holds of learning disabled children. *British Journal of Occupational Therapy,* **41**, No. 8, 282–3.

Penso, D.E. (1987) *Occupational Therapy for Children with Disabilities,* pp. 64–73, Croom Helm, London.

Penso, D.E. (1990) *Keyboard, Graphic and Handwriting Skills: Helping People with Motor Disabilities,* pp. 60–9, 86–9, 95–147, Chapman and Hall, London.

Pickard, P. and Alston, J. (1985) *Helping Secondary School Pupils with Handwriting: Current Research, Identification and Assessment, Guidance,* L.D.A. Wisbech, Cambs, UK.

Pinckney, C. (1989) *Callanetics,* Guild Publishing, London.

Plomer, W. (1950) A Ticket for the Reading Room in *The Penguin Book of Contemporary Verse* Selected by Allott, K., p. 135, Penguin Books, London.

Priestley, J.B. (1946) Bright Day, in *The Concise Oxford Dictionary of Proverbs* compiled by John Simpson, p. 82, Oxford University Press, Oxford.

Riley, J.W. (1899) An Impetuous Resolve in *Riley Child-Rhymes with Hoosier Pictures*, p. 95, The Bowen-Merrill Company, Indianapolis and Kansas City.

Roberts, B.L. Marlow, N. and Cooke, R.W.I. (1989) Motor problems among children of very low birth weight, *British Journal of Occupational Therapy*, **52**, No. 3, 97–9.

Roussounis, S.H., Gaussen, T.H. and Stratton, P. (1987) A 2-year follow-up study of children with motor coordination problems identified at school entry age, *Child: Care, Health and Development*, **13**, 377–91.

Rutter, M. (1989) 'Pathways from childhood to adult life.'*Journal of Child Psychology and Psychiatry*, **30**, No. 1, 23–51.

Sassoon, R. (1983) *The Practical Guide to Children's Handwriting*, Thames and Hudson, London.

Sassoon, R. (1990) *Handwriting: A new persepective*, pp. 4–6. Stanley Thorne, UK.

Sassoon, R. and Briem, G.S.E. (1984) *Teach Yourself Handwriting* Hodder and Stoughton (Educational Department), London.

Shaffer, D. (1978) Soft neurological signs and later psychiatric disorder – a review. *Journal of Child Psychology and Psychiatry*, **19**, 63–5.

Shaffer, D., Schonfeld, I., O'Connor, P.A. *et al.* (1985) Neurological soft signs. Their relationship to psychiatric disorder and intelligence in childhood and adolescence, *Archives of General Psychiatry*, **42**, 342–51.

Sheard, J. (1991) Del boy image seldom works, *Sunday Express*, 11th August, p. 24.

Shelley, E.M. and Riester, E. (1972) Syndrome of minimal brain damage in young adults, *Diseases of the Nervous System*, **33**, 335–8.

Sheridan, M.D. (1975) *From Birth to Five Years*, NFER-Nelson Publishing, London.

Simpson, J. (1985) *The Concise Oxford Dictionary of Proverbs*, p. 179, Oxford University Press, Oxford.

Stephenson, E., McKay, C. and Chesson, R. (1990) An investigative study of early developmental factors in children with motor/learning difficulties, *British Journal of Occupational Therapy*, **53**, No. 1, 4–6.

Stoppard, M. (General ed.) (1980) *The Face and Body Book*, Frances Lincoln, London.

Taylor, J. (1987) Monitoring writing speed, *Handwriting Review*, No. 1, pp. 10–13.

Wallis-Myers, P. (1987) The Sloping Board, *Handwriting Review*, No. 1, 43.

Wood, P.H.N. (1980) Appreciating the consequences of disease: the international classification of impairments, disabilities and handicaps, *WHO Chronicle*, **34**, 376–80.

Further reading

Abbie, M. (1978) Physical treatment for clumsy children, not enough, *Physiotherapy*, **54**, No. 7.

Alston, J. and Taylor, J. (1985) *Helping Left Handed Children with Handwriting*, LDA, Wisbech, Cambs, UK.

Bairstow, P.J. and Laszlo, J.I. (1981) Kinesthetic sensitivity to passive movements and its relationship to motor development and control, *Developmental Medicine and Child Neurology*, **23**, 606–16.

Bishop, D.V.M. (1980) 'Handedness, clumsiness and cognitive ability' *Developmental Medicine and Child Neurology* **22**, 569–79.

Blakemore, C. (1977) *Mechanics of the Mind. BBC Reith Lectures 1976*, Cambridge University Press, Cambridge and London.

Blakemore, C. (1988) *The Mind Machine*, BBC Books, London.

Burr, L.A. (1980) Use of vision in the function of hand eye co-ordination, *British Journal of Occupational Therapy* **43**, No. 2, 59–63.

Chapman, L.J., Lewis, A. and Wedell, K. (1970) A note on reversals in the writing of eight-year-old children, *Remedial Education* **5**, No. 2, 91–4.

Clark, M.M. (1974) *Teaching Left-handed Children*, Hodder and Stoughton, London.

Cratty, B.J. (1973) *Teaching Motor Skills* Prentice-Hall, Englewood Cliffs, New Jersey.

Critchley, M. (1968) Dysgraphia and other anomalies of written speech, *The Paediatric Clinics of North America. Disorders of Motility and Language* **15**, No. 3, 639–50.

Developmental Learning Materials (1976) *Diagnosing and Teaching Scissors Skills* Taskmaster Ltd, Leicester, UK.

Elliot, J.M., Connolly, K.J. and Doyle, A.J.R. (1988)

Development of kinesthetic sensitivity and motor performance in children, *Developmental Medicine and Child Neurology*, **30**, No. 1, 80–92.

Fairgrave, E.M. (1989) Alternative means of assessment: a comparison of standardised tests identifying minimal cerebral dysfunction, *British Journal of Occupational Therapy* **52**, No. 3, 88–92.

Farnham-Diggory, S. (1978) *Learning Disabilities*, Fontana Open Books, London.

Fowler, M.S., Riddell, P.M. and Stein, J.F. (1990) Vergence eye movement control and spatial discrimination in normal and dyslexic children, *Perspectives on Dyslexia*, Vol. 1, pp. 253–73.

Fraser, B.C. (1980) The meaning of handicap in children, *Child: Care, Health and Development*, **6**, No. 2, 83–91.

Gordon, N. and McKinlay, I. (eds) (1980) *Helping Clumsy Children*, Churchill Livingstone, Edinbrough.

Grimley, A.M.D. (1977) *The Clumsy Child*, The Association of Paediatric Physiotherapists.

Hawkins, S. and Gadsby, M. (1991) Perceptuo-motor deficit: A major learning difficulty, *British Journal of Occupational Therapy* **54**, No. 4, 145–9.

Hoare, D. and Larking, D. (1991) Kinesthetic abilities of clumsy children, *Developmental Medicine and Child Neurology*, **33**, No. 8, 671–8.

Horak, R.B., Shumway-Cook, A., Crowe, T. K. and Black, F.O. (1988) Vestibular function and motor proficiency of children with impaired hearing, or with learning disability and motor impairments, *Developmental Medicine and Child Neurology*, **30**, No. 1, 64–79.

Hulme, C., Smart, A., Moran, G. and Mackinlay, I. (1984) Visual, kinesthetic and cross-modal judgements of length by clumsy children: a comparison with young normal children. *Child: Care, Health and Development*, **10**, 117–25.

Inglis, S. (1990) Are there schoolchildren in Lewisham who are experiencing practical difficulties at home and/or school? *British Journal of Occupational Therapy*, **53**, No. 4, 151–4.

Jarman, C. (1977) *The Development of Handwriting Skills: A Resource Book for Teachers*, Basil Blackwell, Oxford.

Kao, H.S. (1973) The effects of hand-finger exercise on human handwriting performance, *Ergonomics*, **16**, 171–5.

Kashani, J.H. (1986) Self-esteem of handicapped children and adolescents, *Developmental Medicine and Child Neurology*, **28**, 77–83.

King-Thomas, L. and Hacker, B.J. (eds) (1987) *A Therapist's Guide to Paediatric Assessment*, Little, Brown and Company, Boston/Toronto.

Kinsbourne, M. (1968) Developmental Gerstmann syndrome, *The Paediatric Clinics of North America. Developmental Disorders of Motility and Language.* **15**, No. 3, 771–8.

Kinsbourne, M., Rufo, D.T., Gamzu, E. *et al.* (1991) Neuro-psychological deficits in adults with dyslexia, *Developmental Medicine and Child Neurology*, **33**, 763–75.

Laszlo, J.I. and Bairstow, P.J. (1980) The measurement of kinesthetic sensitivity in children and adults, *Developmental Medicine and Child Neurology*, **22**, 454–64.

Lazarus, J.C. and Todor, J.I. (1987) Age differences in magnitude of associated movement, *Developmental Medicine and Child Neurology*, **29**, 726–33.

Levy, J. and Reid, M. (1976) Variations in writing posture and cerebral organisation, *Science* **194**, 337–9.

Lord, R. and Hulme, C. (1987) Kinaesthetic sensitivity of normal and clumsy children, *Developmental Medicine and Child Neurology*, **29**, 720–5.

Maclean, M.F. (1991) Parents as co-therapists for children with motor-learning difficulties: a review of the literature, *British Journal of Occupational Theray*, **54**, No. 2, 65–8.

Maclean, M.F. and Chesson, R. (1991) Factors affecting parents' role as co-therapists: a pilot study of parents of children with motor-learning difficulties, *British Journal of Occupational Therapy*, **54**, No. 7, 262–6.

O'Hare, A.E. and Brown, J.K. (1989) Childhood dysgraphia. Part 1. A study of hand function. *Child: Care, Health and Development*, **15**, 79–104.

O'Hare, A.E. and Brown, J.K. (1989) Childhood dysgraphia; Part 2. A study of hand function, *Child: Care, Health and Development.* **15**, 151–66.

Philip & Tracey Ltd (distributor) (1989) *Write Angle: The Desk Top Writing Aid*, Philograph Publications.

Robinson, R.O, Lippold, T. and Land, R. (1986) Body schema: does it depend on bodily-derived sensations? *Developmental Medicine and Child Neurology*, **28**, No. 1, 49–52.

Shafer, S. Q., Stokman, C.J, Shaffer, D. *et al.* (1986) Ten-year consistency in neurological test performance of children without focal neurological defecit. *Developmental Medicine and Child Neurology*, **28**, 417–27.

Smith, P. (1984) Handwriting and spelling, *Gnosis*, No. 5, 24–5.

Springer, S.P. and Deutsch, G. (1989) *Left Brain, Right Brain*, 3rd edn, W.H. Freeman, New York.

Stephenson, E. and McKay, C. (1989) A support group for parents of children with motor-learning difficulties, *British Journal of Occupational Therapy*, **52**, No. 5, 181–3.

Stokman, C.F., Shafer, S. Q., Shaffer, D. *et al.* (1986) Assessment of neurological 'soft signs' in adolescents: reliability studies, *Developmental Medicine and Child Neurology*, **28**, 428–39.

Szatmari, P. and Taylor, D.C. (1984) Overflow movements and behaviour problems: scoring and using a modification of Fog's test. *Developmental Medicine and Child Neurology*, **26**, 297–310.

Touwen, B.C.L. (1972) Laterality and dominance, *Developmental Medicine and Child Neurology*, **14**, 747–55.

Valentine, C.W. (1956) *The Normal Child and Some of His Abnormalities*, Penguin Books, London.

Van der Meulen, J.H.P., Denier Van der Gon, J.J., Gielen, C.C.A.M., Gooskens, R.H.J.M. and Willemse, J. (1991) Visuomotor performance of normal and clumsy children. 11. Arm-tracking with and without visual feedback, *Developmental Medicine and Child Neurology*, **33**, 118–29.

Varma, V. (1984) *Anxiety in Children*, Croom Helm, Kent, UK.

Vernon, M.D. (1971) *The Psychology of Perception*, Penguin Books, London.

Wolff, P.H., Gunnoe, C.E. and Cohen, C. (1983) Associated movements as a measure of developmental age. *Developmental Medicine and Child Neurology*, **25**, 417–29.

Ziviani, J. (1982) Children's prehension while writing, A pilot study, *British Journal of Occupational Therapy*, **45**, No. 9, 306–7.

Appendix A

Glossary of medical and paramedical terms

Abduction: Movement of a limb away from the mid-line of the body.

Adduction: Movement of a limb towards the mid-line of the body.

Agnosia: The inability to recognize and interpret sensory information. Usually 'agnosia' is qualified by the type of inability being described. e.g. Tactile agnosia is the inability to recognize common objects by touch. Visual agnosia is difficulty in recognizing familiar objects and/or people by sight. These inabilities occur despite there being no deficit in the relevant sense organ; the agnosias arise because of the difficulty with interpreting the information which has been received.

Apraxia: Inability to perform certain movements because of lack of ability to plan movements prior to their execution where there is no sensory or motor impairment.

Associated movement: Unintended movement which accompanies an intended movement. e.g. A young child attempting to walk on the outsides of the feet may reflect the position adopted by the feet in the hands. The presence of associated movement normally decreases with increasing age and maturity.

Ataxia: Unsteadiness due to lesions of the cerebellum. Movements are jerky and unsteady, poorly graded and misdirected. Often there are difficulties with posture, balance and orientation in space.

Balance reactions: Compensatory movements or shifts in

muscle tone which occur automatically in order to maintain equilibrium of the body.

Cerebellar lesion: Damage or injury to the cerebellum, the part of the brain which refines coordination of movement. Lesions in this area of the brain may result in ataxia, tremor and/or speech disorders.

Cerebral: Concerning the brain.

Cerebral palsy: A group of disorders in which there is disturbance of movement, paralysis, weakness or incoordination as a result of brain damage.

Clumsy children: Such children 'have severe and specific problems in developing adequate skills of movement, in the absence of general sensory and intellectual handicaps, and do not show signs of overt neurological damage.' (Hulme and Lord, 1986)

Congenital: Existing at or before birth.

Coordination: The patterning of the action of muscles so that they work together to maintain posture, balance and the execution of movements.

Developmental delay: Lateness in the acquisition of skills and abilities compared with the average pattern of development.

Disability: Restriction or lack (resulting from an impairment) of ability to perform an activity in the manner or within the range considered normal for a human being (Wood, 1980).

Distal: Furthest from the centre of the body, the opposite of proximal.

Dysarthria: Difficulty with articulation resulting from impairment of neuromuscular control.

Dysdiadochokinesis: Difficulty with performing rapid reciprocal movements in a rhythmical fashion. e.g. difficulty with rhythmical clapping of the hands or rapid pronation and supination of the hands.

Dysfunction: Difficulty with or impairment of a physical or mental function.

Dysgraphia: Retarded development or abnormality in the skill of handwriting which may occur in addition to poor penmanship or difficulty with one or more aspects of written language.

Dysmorphic: Refers to the malformation of part of the body.

Dyspraxia: Difficulty with planning movement at a cerebral level. There is no loss of power or control of movement but of planning and initiating movement.

Dystonia: Disturbance of muscle tone causing uncontrolled writhing movements.

Eversion: Movement of the foot in which its medial border is depressed and its lateral border is raised.

Extension: The movement of stretching out a part of the body.

Fine motor: Relating to precise movement usually of the hands.

Flexion: Bending of a part of the body; the opposite of extension.

Gait: the manner of walking or running.

Gross motor: Relating to large movements of the body and limbs.

Handicap: A disadvantage for a given individual, resulting from an impairment or a disability, that limits or prevents fulfilment of a role that is normal (depending on age, sex and social and cultural factors) for that individual (Wood, 1980).

Hyperactivity: Overactivity; activity at a higher level than is usually observed. The term is usually applied to children. Some children behave in a hyperactive manner only in certain situations. Parents have been known to describe their child as hyperactive when s/he is really a normally active child.

Hypotonia: Low muscle tone which often results in a degree of floppiness.

Interphalangeal: Between the phalanges, the three bones of the fingers and toes.

IQ (Intelligence Quotient) A means of measuring intellectual ability which is determined by dividing the mental age of a person by chronological age and multiplying by a hundred.

$$\text{e.g.} \qquad \frac{\text{mental age 7.5. years}}{\text{chronological age 10.0 years}} \times 100 = \text{IQ } 75$$

Kinesthesis: The sense which conveys information about the position of the body and limbs; about the direction and extent of movement; the speed of movement; and the force the muscles exert (Laszlo, Bairstow, and Bartrip, 1988).

Kyphosis: An abnormal postural curve of the spin resulting in a humpbacked appearance.

Lateral: Relating to the sides of the body.

Medial: Situated in the middle or towards the middle of the body, the opposite of lateral.

Metacarpo-phalangeal joints: These are formed by the heads of the metacarpals and the bases of the proximal phalanges. These joints form the knuckles of the hand.

Motor: Movement, usually related to muscles or the ennervation of such muscles.

Neurological: Pertaining to nerves.

Neurological soft sign: This 'is a particular form of deviant performance on a motor or sensory test in the neurological status examination. The designation *soft* is usually taken to indicate that the person with the sign shows no other feature of fixed or transient neurological lesion or disorder.' (Shaffer *et al.*, 1985)

Occupational therapy: The treatment of physical and psychiatric conditions through specific activities in order to help people reach their maximum level of function and independence in all aspects of daily life.

Orthoptist: A person who diagnoses anomolies of binocular vision, strabismus and monocular functional amblyopia and administers non-operative treatment (Millidot, 1986).

Pathological: Abnormal.

Perceptual skills: The ability to process, organize and interpret information sensations from internal and external stimuli. e.g. The visual stimulus of seeing a shape with four right angles and four equal sides would normally be perceived as a square.

Perinatal: Relating to the period before, during and shortly after birth.

Peripheral: On the outside, away from the centre.

Phalanges: The bones of the fingers and toes.

Physiotherapy: Treatment of disease, disability or injury by physical means most usually by active methods requiring the cooperation of the person being treated. It is concerned with the maintenance of posture and active movement.

Prognosis: A forecast of the likely outcome of a disease or disability.

Prone: Lying face downwards.

Pronation: Turning the palm of the hand downwards.

Proprioception: Awareness of posture, balance and position. This is due to receptors (called proprioceptors) located within muscles, tendons, joints and the vestibular apparatus of the inner ear (Millidot, 1986).

Proximal: Nearest to the centre of the body, the opposite of distal.

Radial: Relating to the radius, the bone which lies along the thumb side of the forearm.

Reflex: An automatic or invariable response to a stimulus.

Sensory: Relating to sensation.

Soft sign: see Neurological soft sign.

Speech and language therapy: The treatment of a person who has a language disorder which may be congenital or acquired. Such disorders include difficulty with comprehension of language, difficulty with expressive language and problems with articulation. Aims may be to facilitate spoken language or to provide an alternative means of communication such as a system of signing. Speech and language therapy also includes the treatment of feeding disorders.

Stereognosis: The ability to recognize the nature of objects, their shape, size or weight, usually by tactile means (*stereo* solid, *gnosis* knowledge).

Supination: Turning upwards, usually referring to the hand when the palm is uppermost.

Supine: Lying on the back with the face upward.

Tone: The degree of tension in a muscle which is normally sufficiently high to resist the pull of gravity so that people may remain upright but not so high as to interfere with movement.

Tremor: Involuntary trembling of voluntary muscles.

Ulnar: Relating to the ulna, the bone on the inner side of the forearm.

Vestibular sense: This involves the perception of spatial movement and spatial orientation of the body as a whole, due to excitation of receptor cells located in the non-auditory labyrinth of the ear (Corso, 1970).

Appendix B

Suppliers of equipment

Biocurve pen	Nottingham Rehab Ltd, 17 Ludlow Hill Road, West Bridgford, Nottingham, NG2 1BR UK; Distributors in USA: Access-Ability, 1307 West 22nd Place, Tulsa, Oklahoma 74107, USA.
Book stands	Nottingham Rehab Ltd, see above
	Fred Sammons Inc, Box 32, Brookfield, Illinois 60513, USA
Chair raisers	Nottingham Rehab Ltd, see above
	Fred Sammons Inc, see above
Cooking tongs	Nottingham Rehab Ltd, see above
	Hardware stores
Cutlery with enlarged handles	Nottingham Rehab Ltd, see above

Desk-top writing aid (sloping writing surface)	Philip & Tacey Ltd, North Way, Andover, Hants, UK.
Dycem, non-slip material	Nottingham Rehab Ltd, see above
	Fred Sammons, Inc, see above
Foam rubber tubing	Nottingham Rehab Ltd, see above
	Fred Sammons, Inc, see above
Frostig developmental test of visual perception	NFER-Nelson, Darville House, 2 Oxford Road East, Windsor, Berkshire S14 1DF, UK.
Frostig programme for individualized training and remedial training in visual perception	NFER-Nelson, see above
Microwriter	The Foundation for Communication for the Disabled, Foundation House 25 High Street, Woking, Surrey GU21 1BW, UK.
Microscribe	The Foundation for Communication for the Disabled, see above
Pencil grips – triangular Stetro-dimpled pencil grips	LDA, Duke Street, Wisbech, Cambs PE13 2AE, UK.

Distributors in USA:
Didax,
Centenial Industrial Park,
5 Fourth Street,
Peabody,
MA 01960, USA.

Ideal School Supply,
11000 South Laverge Avenue,
Oak Lawn, Illinois 60453, USA.

and Lake Shore,
2695 East Dominguez Street,
P.O. Box 6261,
Carson,
California 90769, USA.

Pencil grips	Taskmaster Ltd, Morris Road, Leicester LE2 6BR, UK.
Plate with lip	Nottingham Rehab Ltd, see above
Scissors (left-handed)	Taskmaster Ltd, see above
	Nottingham Rehab Ltd, see above
	Early Learning Centres
Scissors (palmar grip)	Peta (Toolcraft) Ltd, Stiron House, Electric Avenue, Westcliff-on-Sea, Essex SS0 9NW, UK.
Scissors (whole-hand grip)	Boots the Chemist, larger branches
	Early Learning Centres
	Taskmaster Ltd, see above
	Nottingham Rehab Ltd, see above
	Fred Sammons Inc, see above
Stencils, clear	Taskmaster Ltd, see above

Appendix C

Addresses of societies

UK

Banstead Place Mobility Centre,
Park Road,
Banstead,
Surrey SM7 3EE, UK.

British Association of Occupational Therapists,
6–8 Marshalsea Road,
Southwark,
London SE1 1HL, UK.

British Dyslexia Institute,
133 Gresham Road,
Staines,
Middlesex TW18 2AJ, UK.

British Orthoptist Society,
Tavistock House North,
Tavistock Square,
London WC1H 9HX, UK.

Chartered Society of Physiotherapists,
14 Bedford Row,
London WC1R 4ED, UK.

College of Speech & Language Therapists,
Harold Poster House,
6 Lechmere Road,
London NW2 5BU, UK.

Handwriting Interest Group,
Janet Tootall, Secretary and Treasurer,
West Hill High School,
Thompson Cross,
Stalybridge,
Cheshire SK15 9RD, UK.

SPOD (The Association to Aid the Sexual and Personal
   Relationships of People with Disability),
286 Camden Road,
London N7 0BJ, UK.

The Dyspraxia Trust,
Stella White,
13 Old Hale Way,
Hitchin, Herts SG5 1XJ, UK.

USA

American Occupational Therapy Association Inc.,
1383 Piccard Drive
Rockville
MD 20850, USA.

American Optometric Association Inc.,
245 N. Lindbergh Boulevard
St. Louis
MO 63141, USA.

American Physical Therapy Association,
1111 N. Fairfax Street
Alexandria,
VA 22314, USA.

American Speech – Language – Hearing Association,
10801 Rockville Pike
Rockville
MD 20852, USA.

Index